ANTIBIOTIC ASSOCIATED DIARRHOEA AND COLITIS

DEVELOPMENTS IN GASTROENTEROLOGY

Peña, A.S., Weterman, I.T., Booth, C.C., Strober W., eds: Recent advances in Crohn's disease
ISBN 90 247 2475 9

Motta, P.M., Didio, L.J.A., eds: Basic and clinical hepatology
ISBN 90 247 2404 X

Rachmilewitz, D., ed.: Inflammatory bowel diseases
ISBN 90 247 2612 3

Fleischer, D., Jensen, D., Bright-Asare, P. eds: Therapeutic laser endoscopy in gastrointestinal disease
ISBN 0 89838 577 6

ANTIBIOTIC ASSOCIATED DIARRHOEA AND COLITIS

The role of Clostridium difficile in gastrointestinal disorders

edited by

S. PETER BORRIELLO
Division of Communicable Diseases
Clinical Research Centre, Harrow
Middlesex, UK

1984 **MARTINUS NIJHOFF PUBLISHERS**
a member of the KLUWER ACADEMIC PUBLISHERS GROUP
BOSTON / THE HAGUE / DORDRECHT / LANCASTER

Distributors

for the United States and Canada: Kluwer Boston, Inc., 190 Old Derby Street, Hingham, MA 02043, USA
for all other countries: Kluwer Academic Publishers Group, Distribution Center, P.O.Box 322, 3300 AH Dordrecht, The Netherlands

Library of Congress Cataloging in Publication Data

Library of Congress Cataloging in Publication Data
Main entry under title:

Antibiotic associated diarrhoea and colitis.

(Developments in gastroenterology)
1. Clostridium difficile. 2. Diarrhea--Microbiology.
3. Colitis--Microbiology. I. Borriello, S. Peter.
II. Series. [DNLM: 1. Antibiotics--Adverse effects.
2. Diarrhea--Etiology. 3. Diarrhea--Microbiology.
4. Colitis--Etiology. 5. Colitis--Microbiology.
6. Clostridium--Pathogenicity. WI 407 A629]
QR201.D4A58 1984 616.3'4470145 83-25092
ISBN 0-89838-623-3

ISBN 0-89838-623-3 (this volume)

PRINTED IN THE NETHERLANDS

CONTENTS

Contributors

FIONA E. BARCLAY, H. N. C., Division of Communicable Diseases, Clinical Research Centre, Harrow, Middlesex, U. K.

S. PETER BORRIELLO, PhD., Division of Communicable Diseases, Clinical Research Centre, Harrow, Middlesex, U. K.

DOUGLAS BURDON, M. R. C. Path., Consultant Microbiologist, The General Hospital, Birmingham, U. K.

ROBERT FEKETY, M. D., Professor of Internal Medicine, Division of Infectious Diseases, University of Michigan Medical School, Ann Arbor, Michigan, U. S. A.

W. LANCE GEORGE, M. D., Assistant Chief, Infectious Disease Section, Wadsworth Medical Center, Los Angeles, California, U. S. A.

DAVID M. LYERLY, Ph. D., Research Associate, Department of Anaerobic Microbiology, Virginia Polytechnic Institute and State University, Blacksburg, Virginia, U. S. A.

INGER FLORIN, PH. D., Department of Bacteriology, Karolinska Institute, Stockholm, Sweden.

PAULINE HONOUR, Division of Communicable Diseases, Clinical Research Centre., Harrow, Middlesex, U. K.

MAURY E. MULLIGAN, M. D., Staff Physician, Infectious Disease Section, Wadsworth Medical Center, Los Angeles, California, U. S. A.

ASHLEY B. PRICE, M. R. C. Path., Consultant Histopathologist, Northwick Park Hospital and Clinical Research Centre, Harrow, Middlesex, U. K.

FRANCIS J. TEDESCO, M. D., Professor of Medicine, Chief, Gastroenterology, Medical College of Georgia, Augusta, Georgia, U. S. A.

MONICA THELESTAM, Ph. D., Assistant Professor, Department of Bacteriology, Karolinska Institute, Stockholm, Sweden.

A. R. WELCH, H. N. C., Division of Communicable Diseases, Clinical Resarch Centre, Harrow, Middlesex, U. K.

TRACY D. WILKINS, Ph. D., Professor of Microbiology, Department of Anaerobic Microbiology, Virginia Polytechnic Institute and State University, Blacksburg, Virginia, U. S. A.

Introduction

In the few years since the discovery of the role of *C. difficile* in antibiotic-associated pseudomembranous colitis, the organism has been shown to be involved in many cases of the whole range of antibiotic-associated gastrointestinal disorders as well as cases of pseudomembranous colitis, and diarrhoea, unrelated to recent antibiotic therapy. As with any new pathogen, the discovery of the role of *C. difficile* in disease was accompanied by a great deal of interest and scientific research. Many of the early problems, such as methods of treatment, were quickly dealt with. The organism has attracted the interest of scientists from a wide variety of disciplines. However, much of the research has raised as many questions as it has answered. The evidence that the disease is an infection and that cross-infection may take place has aroused the interests of those involved in epidemiology and hospital infection, and the fact that in the majority of cases, disruption of the normal gut flora must take place before infection will occur has attracted workers interested in microbial interactions and gut ecology. The recent discovery of a second toxin produced by *C. difficile* has added yet another facet to this interesting organism and has given added stimulus to researchers in the field of microbial protein toxins. The recent research into the actions of *C. difficile* toxins is opening up new perspectives in both toxinology and basic cell biology, and it is hoped that the cytotoxin will provide a powerful new tool for the study and understanding of the factors involved in the complicated regulation of the structure and function of cellular microfilaments.

In this book an attempt has been made to collate the information available on all the different aspects of C. difficile and the gastrointestinal diseases associated with it. It is hoped that the information presented will be of value to both the experienced researcher familiar with C. difficile as well as someone in the laboratory contemplating isolation of the organism, or detection of its toxins, for the first time. Above all, I hope that the information presented will also highlight the many areas in which we know very little or nothing, and will, therefore, stimulate interest in this exciting new area of microbiology.

S. P. BORRIELLO

CHAPTER 1

ANTIBIOTICS ASSOCIATED WITH CLOSTRIDIUM DIFFICILE MEDIATED DIARRHOEA AND/OR COLITIS

F. J. TEDESCO

INDEX

Antibiotics Associated with Clostridium difficile Mediated Diarrhea and/or Colitis

F.J. Tedesco

Introduction

Diarrheal complications of antibiotics are among the most common adverse drug reactions encountered in medical practice. With the wider utilization of endoscopic evaluation of the diarrheal illnesses associated with antibiotic usage, patients were noted to have a wide range of endoscopic findings. The spectrum ranged from normal colonic mucosa or non-specific mucosal edema to pseudomembranous colitis (PMC). Although pseudomembranous inflammaton of the intestine predates the antibiotic era and is reported to be caused by chemical poisons, ischemia and recent abdominal surgery, PMC is now a readily accepted and well documented complication of antimicrobial administration (Tedesco, et al. 1974a,b, Bartlett and Gorbach 1977). In the early 1970s, several major theories were being advanced to explain antibiotic associated colitis: direct toxic action of the antibiotic, a change in the bacterial flora, and superinfection by some pathogen or a combination of these factors (Alpers 1978). In the mid-seventies, investigators both in animals and humans implicated Clostridium difficile as an etiologic agent in most cases of antibiotic associated pseudomembranous colitis and 20-30% of antibiotic associated diarrheas in which there was no documented pseudomembrane formation (Larson and Price 1977, Bartlett et al. 1978a, Larson et al. 1978, Bartlett et al. 1977c, Bartlett 1979, George et al. 1978a). A significant breakthrough in the laboratory and clinical evaluation of antibiotic associated diarrhea occurred when it was demonstrated that tissue culture assays of stool from hamsters and humans with antibiotic associated colitis demonstrated a cytopathic change which could be neutralized by clostridial antitoxin. Utilizing the tissue culture assay as well as the endoscopic evaluation of the rectum and colon, a significant amount of data concerning various antibiotics implicated in patients' diarrheal illnesses has been obtained.

It now appears that the offending antibiotics alter the normal balance of the bowel flora. This normal bowel flora contains one or more components which presumably suppresses C. difficile and prevents colonization of the large intestine by this organism (see Ch. 8). The offending antibiotics, by suppressing these competing organisms, allow the C. difficile to colonize the bowel. This entire concept seems reasonable and simple, but an awareness of antibiotic susceptibility test on isolates of

C. difficile is necessary before a clearer picture of this dynamic and complex situation can be brought into focus. The bacteriostatic and bacteriocidal activities of 24 antimicrobial agents toward fifteen isolates of C. difficile were critically evaluated (Fekety et al. 1979). That study demonstrated that rifampin, metronidazole and vancomycin were the most active agents; they inhibited and killed all isolates at concentrations of <2.0 ug/ml. Penicillin G and ampicillin were only slightly less active and drugs such as methicillin, nafcillin, carbenicillin, and tricarcillin were also quite effective at clinically attainable levels. Almost all isolates were inhibited by ≤ 25 ug of cefamandole, cephalothin and cefazolin. Concentrations of ≥ 12.5 ug/ml of cefoxitin or clindamycin were required for inhibition of most isolates. These data dramatically demonstrate that the very same antibiotics which appear to inhibit or kill the C. difficile organism at obtainable concentrations are well documented offending antibiotics in patients with antibiotic associated pseudomembranous colitis.

Antibiotics associated.

Although most reported cases of antibiotic associated pseudomembranous colitis have been related to treatment with clindamycin, lincomycin, ampicillin, or the cephalosporins, almost all other antibiotics (Table 1)

Table 1

Antimicrobials reported to be associated with pseudomembranous colitis in humans

Amoxicillin	Gentamicin
Ampicillin	Kanamycin
Amphotericin	Lincomycin
Carbenicillin	Metronidazole
Cefazolin	Nafcillin
Cefuroxine	Neomycin
Cephalexin	Penicillin G
Cephaloridine	Penicillin V
Cephalothin	Rifampin
Chloramphenicol	Sulfmethoxazole
Clindamycin	Tetracycline
Cloxacillin	Tobramycin
Erythromycin	Trimethoprim
Flucloxacillin	5-Fluorocytosine

have been implicated. In fact, with the possible exception of vancomycin and less so with the aminoglycosides, all antimicrobials should be considered as potentially offending antibiotics with respect to antibiotic associated pseudomembranous colitis in humans (Bartlett 1981b, Borriello and Larson 1981). However, the more frequent antibiotics implicated in colitis associated with Clostridium difficile toxin are listed in Table 2.

Table 2

More frequent antibiotics implicated in colitis associated with Clostridium Difficile toxin

	Time Period	
	pre-1979	post-1979
Clindamycin/Lincomycin	52%	16%
Ampicillin/Amoxacillin	31%	33%
Cephalosporins	9%	30%
Penicillins other than ampicillin/amoxacillin	4%	3%
Other single antibiotics	4%	18%

This table presents the changing incidence of the more frequently implicated antimicrobials in antibiotic associated colitis during two periods of observation. The relative incidence of clindamycin/lincomycin implicated in 1977-1979 was substantially higher than during the 1979-1982 period. Possible explanations for this change in prevalence are that clindamycin/lincomycin associated colitis was the subject of extensive publicity and scrutiny as well as the fact that the usage of clindamycin/lincomycin has decreased as compared to the earlier period. Ampicillin/amoxacillin appears to account for relatively the same percentage of patients with antibiotic associated colitis in the latter period of observation as compared to the initial period. The incidence of cephalosporins being reported as the offending antibiotic has increased. This may be related to the awareness of their potential association with colitis and the increased usage of the stool toxin assay. The increased availability of the tissue culture assay for stool toxin as well as physician awareness that almost any antibiotic can be associated with colitis probably accounts for the increased incidence of "other antibiotics" noted in the latter period of observation.

Now that it is clear that almost any antibiotic regardless of its ability to inhibit or destroy the C.difficile organism can be associated with antibiotic associated pseudomembranous colitis, we should address the following questions: whether or not the route of administration of the antibiotics makes any difference in the occurrence of antibiotic associated colitis, when in the course of therapy does antibiotic diarrhea and colitis occur, and does the amount or total dosage of the antibiotic received by the patient play any role in the occurrence of antibiotic associated pseudomembranous colitis.

1. Route of Administration (Table 3)

Prior to 1974, most reports implicated the development of colitis with the oral administration of the offending antibiotic. In 1974, a prospecive evaluation of patients with clindamycin associated colitis demonstrated that although the development of pseudomembranous colitis was more commonly associated with orally administered clindamycin, pseudomembranous colitis could also occur with intravenous and intramuscular administration of the antibiotic (Tedesco et al.1974a). From the data on Table 3, it appears that the occurrence of pseudomembranous colitis occurred four times more frequently with the oral route of administration than the parenteral route of administration of the clindamycin. These data have been validated with many other antimicrobial agents, and it appears that although pseudomembranous colitis does occur with both the oral and parenterally administered antibiotics, it appears to occur two to four times more frequently with the orally administered antibiotics.

Table 3

Clindamycin: Route of administration

Route	Total number of patients	Number of patients with pseudomembranous colitis
Oral	80	13
Intravenous	72	2
Intramuscular	3	1

2. Development of Diarrhea and Colitis (Tedesco et al. 1974a, Tedesco 1976).

In the same study it was demonstrated that although most patients developed their onset of diarrhea and colitis within the fourth to ninth day while they were receiving the antibiotic therapy, some patients developed the onset of diarrhea and pseudomembranous colitis days to weeks after completing a full and uneventful course of the antibiotic. The majority of patients who develop pseudomembranous colitis after completing their course of antibiotics develop their diarrhea and colitis within the first five days after therapy. Unfortunately patients have been seen to develop diarrhea and pseudomembranous colitis as late as six weeks after receiving a course of antibiotics. Whether these patients had truely antibiotic associated pseudomembranous colitis or spontaneously occurring pseudomembranous colitis remains unanswered.

3. Dosage of antibiotic (Tedesco et al. 1974a)

Table 4 summarizes the total dosage of antibiotics received by 102 patients with antibiotic associated pseudomembranous colitis. From these data, it appears that the occurrence of antibiotic associated colitis is not dose dependent. Patients have been seen who have developed diarrhea and pseudomembranous colitis after receiving only one or two doses (500 milligrams or less) of an antibiotic, while other patients have received greater than 20 grams of an antibiotic without developing diarrhea or pseudomembranous colitis.

Table 4

Antibiotic dosage in patients with antibiotic associated pseudomembranous colitis

Total antibiotic dose in grams	Number of patients with pseudomembranous colitis
Less than 1	6
1 to 3.9	28
4 to 9.9	36
10 to 20	28
Greater than 20	4

In summary, it appears that nearly all drugs with an antibacterial spectrum of activity may be considered as a potential cause of C.difficile induced pseudomembranous colitis. The route of administration, the completion of an uneventful course of the antibiotic, or the antibiotic's known ability to inhibit or kill the C.difficile organism play little predictive value in allowing the clinician to define the patient who will develop antibiotic associated pseudomembranous colitis.

CHAPTER 2

SPECTRUM OF DISEASE

D. W. BURDON

INDEX

SPECTRUM OF DISEASE

D. W. BURDON

INTRODUCTION

Antibiotic-associated pseudomembranous colitis (PMC) is an acute disorder affecting the colonic and rectal mucosa. The mucosal lesions may be distributed throughout the entire length of the colon and rectum, or they may be confined to one or more localised areas. Diarrhoea is the most characteristic symptom. When Clostridium difficile was first identified as a cause of PMC in humans (Bartlett et al., 1978a, George, R.H. et al., 1978, George et al., 1978c, Larson et al., 1978), the presence of the organism and its cytotoxin in the faeces of affected patients appeared to offer a simple and reliable method of diagnosis for a distinct clinical entity. Subsequent experience has shown that the spectrum of disease caused by C. difficile extends far beyond patients with PMC to include some patients with antibiotic-associated diarrhoea.

C. difficile has also been suspected to have a role in other disorders, notably in the newborn in whom it readily colonises the intestinal tract, and in patients with chronic inflammatory bowel disease. It is occasionally encountered in infected wounds and in the immunosuppressed patient it appears to be responsible for a distinct syndrome.

PSEUDOMEMBRANOUS COLITIS

This was the first disease to be attributed to C. difficile and is the most important in terms of morbidity and mortality. The clinical features are variable and have been described by Tedesco (1976), Bartlett and Gorbach (1977), Kappas et al. (1978) and Mogg et al. (1979). The principal symptom is watery diarrhoea which occurs in nearly all cases. In most patients the frequency of diarrhoea is between 3 and 8 times daily but may be greater (Mogg et al. 1979). The diarrhoea is typically watery, is not usually offensive and often contains excess mucus, but no grossly visible pus or blood. Although the faeces are not usually bloodstained, tests for occult blood are commonly positive. Bloody diarrhoea has been estimated to occur in 10% of patients (Tedesco, 1982a), but in the large series reported by Mogg et al. (1979) it was never observed, and in his earlier report, Tedesco (1976) described bloody diarrhoea in only one of 47 patients. Another form of acute colitis must be distinguished from PMC in patients who have bloody diarrhoea. Typically there is a profuse watery diarrhoea which becomes grossly bloody in 12-24 hours. On endoscopy, the patients have a normal rectum and sigmoid colon, but have erythematous friable segments of mucosa on the right side of the colon principally at the hepatic flexure. C. difficile and its cytotoxin are not associated with this right-sided haemorrhagic colitis which usually follows oral penicillin or ampicillin therapy (Toffler et al. 1978, Sakurai et al. 1979).

Most patients with PMC develop diarrhoea 4-9 days after the start of antibiotic therapy and sometimes while they are still receiving antibiotics. In 25-40% of patients the onset may be delayed for 2-10 weeks (Tedesco, 1982a). The development of pseudomembranes may be delayed for a variable time after the onset of diarrhoea. Occasional fatal cases of PMC have been diagnosed at post-mortem in patients who did not have diarrhoea.

In patients who have not been given specific therapy, the duration of symptoms may be as short as 48 hours or as long as 50 days, but in the majority of patients resolution of symptoms is complete within 10-14 days of stopping antibiotics (Tedesco, 1976).

Many patients complain of cramping hypogastric pain before or coinciding with the onset of diarrhoea. In some, the combination of abdominal pain, rebound tenderness, a leucocytosis and fever may mimic an acute surgical abdomen and such symptoms may occur in 10-20% of patients (Tedesco, 1982a). Toxic megacolon is a rare complication. Nausea and vomiting may also accompany the diarrhoea in a few cases.

A low grade fever which rarely exceeds 39.5°C is common. Mogg et al. (1979) found that 40 (66%) of their 60 patients had a fever greater than 37.5°C, and of these 18 (26%) had a fever greater than 38.5°C. The same authors documented white cell counts varying from 9 to 60 x 10^9/l and exceeding 15.0 x 10^9/l in 40% of their patients.

The fully developed mucosal lesions of the colon and rectum form discrete elevated plaques. These are composed of fibrinous exudate containing epithelial and cellular debris, and are separated by normal or relatively normal mucosa which may be covered by mucus. A variable appearance is seen in the size, extent and distribution of the plaques. Typically, they vary in size from a few millimetres to 2 centimetres in diameter, but in severe cases they may coalesce to form a semi-confluent pseudomembrane. In some patients the only macroscopic evidence of colitis is oedema with or without a friable mucosa, but in these cases histological examination will often reveal the early lesions of PMC. Tedesco (1979) performed colonoscopy on 6 patients who had laboratory evidence of colitis from the presence of C. difficile cytotoxin in their stools, but in whom sigmoidoscopy was normal. Five of these 6 patients demonstrated pseudomembranes in various areas of the colon. Two patients had lesions in the caecal area, ascending colon and hepatic flexure. Two further patients had similar lesions with additional lesions in the transverse colon. The fifth patient had pseudomembranes only at the splenic flexure. In a similar investigation, 11 (85%) of 13 patients in whom colonoscopy was done had lesions confined to the colon (Seppala et al. 1981). The same authors commented that most published cases of severe PMC and one of their own patients who died had involvement of the sigmoid colon and rectum. This supports the idea that the extent and location of the mucosal damage is related to the severity and duration of the disease. Further evidence for this is given by a study comparing patients with faecal cytotoxin and rectal PMC with a group of patients with faecal cytotoxin and a normal rectal mucosa. The duration of diarrhoea was significantly longer in those with rectal pseudomembrane (Burdon et al., 1981). The distribution of lesions is also of interest in connection with reports of PMC published before the introduction of antibiotic therapy. Cases without antecedent antibiotic use do occur but are uncommon (Peikin et al., 1980, Wald et al., 1980). Formerly, they were seen most often following gastrointestinal surgery, but it is uncertain whether they were all cases of C. difficile-associated PMC because they included patients with lesions of the small intestine, and even of the stomach and oesophagus as well as the colon and rectum (Pettet et al., 1954). It is possible that another aetiology such as ischaemic colitis was responsible for these atypical cases. Ischaemic colitis is recognised as a distinct entity, although it may be difficult to distinguish histologically in its advanced form (Price and Davies, 1977). The similarity between PMC and ischaemic colitis raises the possibility that the two disorders share in part a common pathogenetic mechanism even though the initiating causes are quite different. If this is correct, one might expect the two disorders to be synergistic or additive. Many clinicians have expressed the opinion that PMC is more common in the elderly, but this might be because of the predominance of this age group in hospital where most cases occur. As a corollary to this, PMC is uncommon in children even though C. difficile is frequently carried in the faecal flora during the first year of life. If not more common in the elderly, PMC is certainly more serious and carries a higher mortality. In the series of patients studied by Price and Davies (1977), PMC was noted to be most serious in the chronically sick or post-operative patients, and all deaths occurred in those over 50 years of age. Likewise, Mogg et al. (1979) observed a mortality rate of 10% in patients under the age of 60 years, and 41% in patients who were more than 60 years of age.

ANTIBIOTIC ASSOCIATED DIARRHOEA

The routine investigation of faeces from patients with antibiotic-associated diarrhoea for the presence of C. difficile and its cytotoxin, has identified many patients with positive findings in one or both of these tests, in whom rectal pseudomembrane is absent. The frequency of this association of C. difficile with antibiotic-induced diarrhoea is variable and ranges from zero up to 15% (Keighley et al., **1978a**) and 34% (George et al., **1982a**). These differences may be related to environment, to the type of antibiotic used and the route of administration, and to the clinical criteria used in selecting patients for investigation. It can not be said with certainty what proportion of these patients have PMC, non-specific colitis or uncomplicated diarrhoea. Previously cited data indicates that most patients with faecal cytotoxin and a normal rectal mucosa have pseudomembranes which can be seen on colonoscopy (Tedesco, 1979, Seppala et al, 1981). However it is likely that the patients in these studies were representative of the more severe end of the spectrum of disease. When all patients with diarrhoea defined as 3 or more bowel actions per day are studied, many are found with cytotoxin in whom the diagnosis of PMC would not have been suspected on clinical grounds, (Mogg et al., 1979). In the latter study, 32 patients were found to have a faecal cytotoxin and of these 21 (66%) had PMC on the basis of sigmoidoscopic appearance and histological examination. Of the remainder, 8 (24%) had non-specific colitis and 3 (10%) had diarrhoea without any rectal abnormality.

It appears therefore that C. difficile might be responsible for some episodes of antibiotic-associated diarrhoea and that non-specific colitis and diarrhoea represent part of a spectrum of disease with PMC as the most florid form. The evidence that C. difficile is involved in this extended spectrum of disease is however incomplete. Price and Davies, (1977) observed similarities between the histological appearances of antibiotic-associated non-specific colitis and PMC. Also, many patients with antibiotic-associated diarrhoea and faecal C. difficile have either a normal mucosa or non-specific colitis which on repeat examination shows progression to pseudomembrane formation (Keighley et al., 1978a). Finally, non-specific colitis and PMC may co-exist in different areas of the mucosa in the same patient. Other data listed in Table 1 also support the concept of a spectrum of disease ranging from PMC to diarrhoea. The faecal cytotoxin titre and duration of diarrhoea are both significantly less in patients without rectal pseudomembranes, and the white cell count is lower.

Table 1. Relation between rectal pseudomembrane and clinical findings in patients with faecal cytotoxin.

	Rectal pseudomembrane		
	Present	Absent	
Faecal cytotoxin titre	n=17	n=11	
Range	100-80,000	100-128,000	
Median	16,000	3,200	*
Duration of diarrhoea (days)	n=14	n=11	
Range	5-50	3-16	
Median	16	6	**
White cell count (x 10^9/l)	n=18	n=14	
Range	9.9-44.4	7.5-18.4	
Median	17.2	10.9	N.S.
Serum albumin (g/l)	n=18	n=16	
Range	22-44	21-46	
Median	29	29.5	N.S.

n = No. of patients　　N.S. = not significant
* P <0.05　　** P <0.005

Despite these observations it can not be assumed that C. difficile is playing a pathogenic role in all patients with diarrhoea in whose faeces cytotoxin is present. The significance of C. difficile without cytotoxin is less certain, even when the organism is shown to produce cytotoxin *in vitro*. In healthy persons C. difficile is only rarely cultured from faeces (George et al., 1978b). After antibiotic therapy it is found more frequently, but not all carriers develop diarrhoea or signs of colitis. In a prospective survey of antibiotic-associated post-operative diarrhoea, C. difficile was isolated from the faeces of 2 of 16 patients who had developed diarrhoea and from 4 of 12 control patients who remained well. Cytotoxin was produced in vitro by all of the C. difficile isolates but it was not detected in the faeces of any of the patients. Lishman et al., (1981a) found faecal cytotoxin in 19% of 53 patients with antibiotic-associated diarrhoea but also in 7.5 % of the same number of antibiotic treated patients who did not have diarrhoea. It is apparent therefore that neither C. difficile nor its cytotoxin are diagnostic for C. difficile-induced disease. The same conclusion was reached by George et al., (1982a) who recovered C. difficile from 6 of 13 individuals, and cytotoxin from 3 of 12 individuals without diarrhoea following antibiotics. They found that the titre of faecal cytotoxin was not appreciably different from that in patients with PMC, non-specific colitis or diarrhoea. The overall conclusion is that patients with diarrhoea as the sole feature of C. difficile-associated illness follow a less severe course than patients with non-specific colitis or PMC, and that the three conditions form a continuous spectrum of illness which in its mildest form merges into and is indistinguishable from normality.

SPORADIC DIARRHOEAL DISEASE

Several groups of investigators have surveyed the incidence of C. difficile in persons with acute onset of diarrhoea acquired in the community. Brettle et al., (1982) recovered C. difficile from 19 of 154 patients, 7 of whom had not taken antibiotics. Only one of these 7 patients had faecal cytotoxin and this was at a very low titre. A salmonella was isolated from 4 of the 12 patients, an association also noticed by others (Nash et al., 1982, Jewkes et al., 1981). These observations are of interest because enteric pathogens have been recognised as a predisposing factor in PMC since before the antibiotic era. In a larger study (Falsen *et al.*, 1980) *C. difficile* was isolated from 81 of 2,390 faecal samples representing 56 patients of whom 43% were children under 4 years of age, and 50 had diarrhoea. In 20 (36%) of these 56 patients, salmonella, campylobacter or yersinia were also found, and antibiotics had been used in less than 48%. These authors proposed that any change in the normal bacterial flora due to causes such as antibiotic therapy or enteric infection, increases the possibility of isolating *C. difficile*. There is little data to suggest that *C. difficile* can behave as a primary enteric infection in such patients. Nevertheless, infection by *C. difficile* does occur in the absence of known precipitating causes (Peikin *et al.*, 1980, Wald *et al.*, 1980), but is uncommon. It remains a possibility that sporadic cases arise as a consequence of infection by an enteric pathogen which is no longer detectable when the faecal specimen is cultured, or by an unknown pathogen (Jewkes *et al.*, 1982).

INFLAMMATORY BOWEL DISEASE

Early in 1980, two reports described an association in patients with chronic inflammatory bowel disease (CIBD), between the presence of *C. difficile* cytotoxin and acute exacerbation of symptoms (LaMont and Trnka, 1980, Bolton *et al.*, 1980). In the first, cytotoxin was described in the faeces of 6 patients during symptomatic relapse. Only 2 of these patients had received antibiotics although a further 2 had received sulphasalazine, a drug which is metabolised by intestinal bacteria to yield active sulphonamide. The second report concerned 24 patients with CIBD and diarrhoea of whom 5 had faecal cytotoxin. Two of these had received sulphasalazine. From this small number of cases it appeared that a slightly larger number of *C. difficile* infections than is usual were occurring without relationship to antibiotic use.

In an enlarged group of patients, LaMont and Trnka (1981) reported the presence of cytotoxin in the stool of 11 (19%) of 59 patients, and of these 4 had no history of exposure to antibiotics or to sulphasalazine. The incidence of a positive cytotoxin test was said to correspond strongly with the activity of the underlying disease, being present in none of 25 mild cases, 2 out of 19 moderate flares and 9 out of 15 severe flares. Vancomycin therapy was given to 8 patients in 5 of whom it was clearly effective. Two other studies reported contrary findings. Meyers et al., (1981), found cytotoxin only in patients who had been exposed to antibiotics within two months, and the presence of cytotoxin did not correlate with disease activity. In a larger series of 74 acute hospital admissions for relapse of CIBD only 4 patients who had all received antibiotics had faecal cytotoxin (Keighley et al., 1981), and the authors concluded that C. difficile is a rare cause of acute exacerbation of Crohn's disease and ulcerative colitis unless patients have been exposed to antibiotics. In the same study, C. difficile was isolated from 11 of 43 specimens from patients whose faeces had been cultured on admission to hospital. Cytotoxin was not detected in any of these patients, and 4 of the C. difficile isolations were not related to antibiotic use. It is possible therefore that the intestinal environment in patients with CIBD provides favourable conditions for colonisation by C. difficile (Dorman et al., 1982). In CIBD the proportion of patients who are culture positive and cytotoxin negative compared with culture and cytotoxin positive is significantly higher than amongst patients with colitis or antibiotic-associated diarrhoea (Burdon et al., 1980). This was noted to be similar to the situation in the newborn infant in whom C. difficile without cytotoxin is a frequent finding and it was suggested that the intestinal milieu of CIBD patients and infants might be unfavourable to toxin production. Another interpretation consistent with epidemiological findings (Burdon, 1982) is the suggestion that most strains of C. difficile are relatively avirulent, and that the pathogenic potential of strains acquired in the community by CIBD patients would be less than that of isolates from a group of patients with colitis which had been mostly acquired in a hospital environment where cross-infection occurs.

If this is true, it might explain the generally low but variable incidence of symptomatic illness caused by C. difficile in CIBD despite a relatively high carriage rate.

Taking an overall view of the available data, it seems that patients with CIBD are subject to secondary infection by C. difficile following antibiotic therapy, and like other individuals experience the whole spectrum of disease ranging from PMC to diarrhoea, as well as an increased tendancy to become asymptomatic carriers. Their response to specific therapy with vancomycin must be judged against a background of chronic symptoms, and is only likely to be dramatic in those with quiescent underlying disease and severe secondary involvement by C. difficile. It seems therefore that C. difficile should be added to the list of organisms such as shigella and campylobacter which can occur as incidental events in individuals already compromised by CIBD and produce a symptomatic episode which might be mistaken for relapse of their underlying chronic disorder.

Another chronic bowel disorder in which a role for C. difficile has been suggested is the irritable bowel syndrome (Tvede and Willumsen, 1982). They reported an increased isolation rate in patients with this condition, but did not declare the antibiotic exposure of their patients. The carriage of detectable C. difficile was of short duration, and these results require confirmation and long-term follow-up of patients to establish the correlation between carriage and clinical status.

CLOSTRIDIUM DIFFICILE IN CHILDREN

C. difficile was first isolated from the faeces of infants by Hall and O'Toole (1935). They demonstrated that it was lethal when injected into guinea-pigs in which it caused convulsions, and speculated that it might account for otherwise unexplained convulsions in infants on the basis of absorption of toxin from the intestinal tract. Snyder (1937) tested this hypothesis by oral challenge of the guinea-pig, rat and dog with toxin containing broth suspensions, and in the absence of any harmful effect concluded that the toxin was not absorbed, and therefore unlikely to be harmful to infants.

More recent observations have confirmed the high carriage rate in neonates of around 40% (Larson et al., 1978). An investigation of 218 children between the ages of 2 weeks and 15 years gave a peak incidence of 64% in children aged 1-8 months, and 4% in children below and above that age range (Holst et al., 1981). No significant difference was observed between carriage rates in children with gastro-enteritis (23%) and those who were well (17%) and no child had clinical evidence of PMC. A high carriage rate of 53% was recorded in children less than one year old by Stark et al., (1982). These authors carried out repeated cultures on groups of 5 breast-fed and 5 formula-fed babies for 32 weeks. Four of the breast-fed and all of the formula-fed babies acquired C. difficile at some time, but the duration of carriage was shorter in the breast-fed than in the formula-fed babies. The finding of Larson et al., (1978) that carriage rates were similar in breast-fed and formula-fed babies is consistent with these results, but cytotoxin data seems to contradict this and may reflect local variations in the opportunities for colonisation (Donta and Myers, 1982). They found faecal cytotoxin in 10.5% of newborn infants mostly between the 3rd and 6th day of life. It was much more common in the neonatal intensive care unit where 55% of neonates were cytotoxin positive. Increased rates of cytotoxin positivity were associated with vaginal delivery and breast feeding. Despite these findings, none of the normal infants with cytotoxin and less than a third of those in the intensive care unit had intestinal symptoms.

The rarity of PMC in neonates and children is surprising in view of the high incidence of C. difficile carriage. Generally however, cytotoxin is absent, or when present occurs at a low titre (Rietra et al., 1978). The reason for the absence of symptomatic illness in children with cytotoxin is unknown. Suggested explanations have included inactivation of toxin by other intestinal micro-organisms, absence of receptors for toxin binding (Viscidi and Bartlett, 1981), and avirulence of most strains of C. difficile (Burdon, 1982). Nevertheless, PMC does occur in neonates (Donta et al., 1981), in infants (Richardson et al., 1981), and in older children (Butts et al., 1977, Viscidi and Bartlett, 1981). The clinical presentation as in adults is highly variable, but virtually all affected children have diarrhoea. Common presenting symptoms are fever, nausea, vomiting and abdominal distension. Of the 5 cases reported by Butts et al., (1977), one was found to have lesions affecting the distal half of the small bowel as well as the colon. They also observed ascites, pleural effusion and peripheral oedema in 4 children who also had low serum albumin levels. Other complications described in children are toxic megacolon and severe dehydration with electrolyte disturbances (Viscidi and Bartlett, 1981). The last authors noted a mortality of 28% in 25 patients collected from the medical literature compared with zero mortality in their own more recent series of 10 cases most of whom were treated with vancomycin.

Children with Hirschsprung's disease appear to be especially prone to develop enterocolitis, and this has been related to C. difficile in 4 of 6 children who had titres of faecal cytotoxin which were well above the range usually found in some normal children. In 2 of these children histological confirmation of PMC was obtained (Thomas et al., 1982).

Involvement of C. difficile in neonatal necrotizing enterocolitis (NEC) has also been suggested (Cashore et al., 1981), but most investigators have discounted this. Cytotoxin was not found in the stool of any of 24 infants with NEC (Bartlett et al., 1978d). Others have found C. difficile and cytotoxin in children with NEC, but the titre of cytotoxin and the frequency of positive findings have not differed from unaffected control children (Sherertz et al., 1982, Smith et al., 1980).

An association between the sudden infant death syndrome (SIDS) and PMC in a 3 month old infant has raised the possibility that C. difficile might be involved in this unexplained cause of sudden infant death (Scopes et al., 1980). This is reminiscent of the previously mentioned suggestion of involvement of *C. difficile* toxin in infantile convulsions, and is improbable for the same reasons, namely that toxin does not appear to be absorbed and can not be detected in serum. Caution in linking SIDS with *C. difficile* has been urged for the same reasons as with NEC, and also because the seasonal incidence of SIDS and its lack of association with antibiotic usage differ from PMC (Cooperstock *et al.*, 1982).

ARTHRITIS AND PMC

An unusual complication of PMC which merits separate consideration is reactive arthritis (Rollins and Moeller, 1976). A recent case report more firmly established the role of *C. difficile* in this arthropathy by demonstrating very high titres of cytotoxin-neutralising antibody in the patient's serum (Fairweather *et al.*, 1980). Similar antibodies could not be found in the sera of 11 other patients with PMC who did not have arthritis. In this patient, diarrhoea had resolved by 10 days, but she remained unwell with fever, leucocytosis, generalised myalgia and arthropathy. Effusions developed in both knees, the shoulder, neck, wrists and ankles were painful, but the small joints of the hands were not involved. The arthritis resolved completely during a period of 3 months. At least two other case reports describing this complication have been published (Bolton *et al.*, 1980, Abbott and Caughey, 1982).

CLOSTRIDIUM DIFFICILE IN NEUTROPENIC PATIENTS

An atypical presentation of *C. difficile* associated disease in which infection was invasive has been described in neutropenic patients with intestinal colonisation by *C. difficile* (Rampling *et al.*, 1982). Gram-positive bacilli were seen in the submucosal tissue of the colon and *C. difficile* was isolated from blood cultures in 2 patients. The identity of the submucosal bacilli was not established but recent unpublished observations by the same authors indicate that *C. septicum* was present. None of the patients had pseudomembranes and only one of 4 had diarrhoea. The absence of pseudomembranes may have resulted from inability to mount a local neutrophil response within the colon, or the infecting *C. difficile* may have lacked the potential to produce this type of lesion. Other characteristic features of the patients were jaundice, renal failure, ascites and acute abdominal symptoms. In the resected colon of one of the patients there was oedema of the mucosa, submucosa and serosa with areas of necrosis. This clinical picture is suggestive of local and systemic toxaemia, and may be attributable to the absence of a normal tissue defensive response to infection. The relative importance of *C. difficile* and *C. septicum* in contributing to this toxaemic state remains to be established.

CLOSTRIDIUM DIFFICILE IN TISSUE INFECTION

C. difficile has been isolated from traumatic and surgical wounds, blood cultures and various other body sites, and most medical laboratories which routinely identify all of their clostridial isolates can expect to see this organism from time to time. Several individual case reports have been reviewed, (Smith and King, 1962). It could not be concluded that *C. difficile* was responsible for death in any of the 3 fatal cases, and in the non-fatal cases there was little to indicate that it was anything other than a secondary invader doing no harm except perhaps locally. A recent case report of chronic osteomyelitis due to *C. difficile* suggests that it may occasionally be a more aggressive pathogen even though signs of systemic toxicity did not occur (Riley and Karthigasu, 1982).

CHAPTER 3

DIAGNOSIS AND TREATMENT OF ANTIMICROBIAL AGENT-ASSOCIATED DIARRHOEA AND COLITIS

W. L. GEORGE

INDEX

DIAGNOSIS AND TREATMENT OF ANTIMICROBIAL AGENT-ASSOCIATED DIARRHEA AND COLITIS

W.L. GEORGE

INTRODUCTION

Since the inception of the antimicrobial era in the late 1930's, diarrhea or colitis has been a relatively frequent, and sometimes serious complication of antimicrobial therapy in humans. For approximately 40 years, the etiology of such diarrhea was not known, although a number of theories were proposed. The lack of understanding of antimicrobial-associated diarrhea by clinicians led to a variety of different therapies, many of which, although without benefit, were potentially harmful. The development of the hamster model of antimicrobial-induced Clostridium difficile ileocecitis has provided a model for the study of antimicrobial-associated diarrhea in humans. Some substantial differences exist between hamsters and humans as regards antimicrobial-induced diarrhea; application of facts gained from study of the animal model of diarrhea, therefore, should be applied to humans with caution. It is known, however, that C. difficile is an important cause of antimicrobial-associated diarrhea in humans and that therapy directed against C. difficile is effective.

DIAGNOSIS OF ANTIMICROBIAL AGENT-ASSOCIATED DIARRHEAS

The approach to the patient with antimicrobial-associated diarrhea requires a search for an etiological agent. Such an evaluation will lead to the implication of C. difficile in an appreciable number of cases (especially the more severe cases of diarrhea); in the majority of instances, however a pathogen will not be found. Occasionally, gram-negative bacillary enteric pathogens (Campylobacter, Salmonella, Shigella or Yersinia), protozoa (Entamoeba histolytica or Giardia lamblia), or Staphylococcus aureus may be the apparent cause of the antimicrobial-associated diarrhea. In order to avoid unnecessary and potentially harmful therapy, the clinician should always ensure that a proper diagnostic evaluation is done.

General approach to the patient with antimicrobial associated diarrhea

The initial evaluation of the patient should include a thorough history and physical examination, and laboratory tests as indicated by the clinical findings (George, 1980). Areas that should be specifically addressed in the evaluation are the severity of the diarrheal illness and the possibility that the diarrhea might not be related to the antimicrobial therapy. Therefore, the following information should be sought: the presence of, and degree of fever; the frequency of bowel movements; the character of the feces (bloody, watery, mucoid, etc.); the presence of abdominal cramps or pain; assessment of the degree of dehydration; the use of medications (other than antimicrobials) that may cause diarrhea; presence of underlying diseases that may be associated with diarrhea; history of recent travel; and history of recent animal exposure.

Microscopic examination of feces has generally not been helpful in evaluation of antibiotic-associated diarrhea; such examinations would, of course, be beneficial in the occasional instance of Campylobacter or protozoal enteritis that might develop in association with antimicrobial therapy.

The need for endoscopy (sigmoidoscopy or colonoscopy) or barium enema examination of the colon for evaluation of antimicrobial-associated diarrhea is controversial (George et al., 1982b; Bartlett, 1982 ; and Tedesco, 1982a). It is reasonable to reserve such tests for situations in which rapid diagnosis is essential for optimal clinical management; the disease process is judged to be severe; or the diagnosis is unclear despite completion of an appropriate noninvasive evaluation. Endoscopy is of value for diagnosis of pseudomembranous colitis (but not other forms of antimicrobial-associated diarrhea) and for diagnosis of potentially confounding illnesses such as amebiasis and the idiopathic inflammatory bowel diseases. In the majority of instances of antimicrobial-associated diarrhea, endoscopy (or barium enema examination of the colon) will alter neither the diagnosis nor the management.

The initial evaluation in addition to the history, physical examination and routine laboratory tests, should include evaluation of a fecal sample for C. difficile.

Diagnosis of C. difficile-induced diarrhea

Several different techniques have been suggested as a means for diagnosis of C. difficile-induced diarrhea; these include detection of C. difficile in feces, detection of colonic plaques or a pseudomembrane, and detection of a product of C. difficile in feces.

A selective medium (CCFA) for recovery of C. difficile from feces has been developed (George et al., 1979c; and George et al., 1982a) and subsequently modified by a number of investigators. Although CCFA is a very sensitive means for detecting C. difficile in feces, the diagnostic value of a positive culture is limited by the presence of asymptomatic intestinal carriers of C. difficile (Viscidi et al., 1981 ; Nakamura et al., 1981a ; and George et al., 1978b). A properly done culture that is negative appears to exclude C. difficile as the cause of diarrhea, whereas a positive culture only indicates that C. difficile might be the cause of diarrhea.

Fluorescent antibody testing (Wilson et al., 1982 b) to demonstrate the presence of C. difficile in feces does not appear to offer any advantage over culture and may be less specific than is culture. Serodiagnosis has not been adequately studied, but would not likely be a useful test for diagnosis because seroconversion does not occur in all patients and because the length of time required for seroconversion to occur would preclude the diagnostic utility of this type of test.

It has been noted that 90% or more of cases of antimicrobial-associated pseudomembranous colitis are due to C. difficile (George et al., 1982b; and Bartlett et al., 1980a). The detection of colonic pseudomembranes in the setting of antimicrobial therapy is very strongly suggestive of, but not diagnostic for C. difficile-induced diarrhea.

Several different products of C. difficile can be detected in the feces. Clostridium difficile in pure culture produces a distinctive pattern of organic and volatile fatty acid end-products (as measured by gas-liquid chromatography); analysis of feces for these end-products as a diagnostic test, however, is fraught with hazard because the bacteria that comprise the normal fecal flora (collectively) are capable of producing the same pattern of metabolic end-products.

Although C. difficile produces at least two distinct toxins (herein termed enterotoxin and cytotoxin), it is not known whether assay for the more recently described enterotoxin (Taylor et al., 1981 ; Banno et al., 1981) will be found to be of diagnostic value.

The best means for diagnosis at this time is detection of the cytotoxin of C. difficile in feces (Bartlett, 1982). Although several investigators have suggested that counterimmunoelectrophoresis of feces for cytotoxin is a useful diagnostic test (Ryan et al., 1980 ; Welch et al., 1980), others have noted serious deficiencies with this type of assay as compared to the tissue culture assay (Poxton and Byrne, 1981b; West and Wilkins, 1982 ; and Levine et al., 1982). The presence of cytotoxin (as measured by the tissue culture assay) in feces correlates well with the presence of C. difficile in feces and the response of diarrhea to specific therapy directed against C. difficile. An excellent description of the tissue culture assay for cytotoxin has been published by one of the groups that discovered the role of C. difficile in diarrhea (Chang et al., 1979a); this assay is recommended to clinical laboratories.

The cytotoxin assay may also occasionally be positive in patients who have diarrhea apparently not related to antimicrobial therapy; these include exacerbation of symptoms of chronic idiopathic inflammatory bowel disease (Meyers et al., 1981 ; Trnka and LaMont, 1981 ; and Bartlett, 1981a), diarrhea related to cancer chemotherapy (Fainstein et al., 1981 ; and Cudmore et al., 1982), and diarrhea of apparently spontaneous onset (Howard et al., 1980 ; Wald et al., 1980 Peikin et al., 1980 ; and Moskovitz and Bartlett, 1981). The detection of cytotoxin in such patients strongly suggests that their diarrhea, (or exacerbation of inflammatory bowel disease) is due to C. difficile.

In contrast to adults, asymptomatic young children and infants are frequently intestinal carriers of C. difficile and may also have cytotoxin present in feces (Viscidi et al., 1981). Because of this, a positive cytotoxin assay is of limited diagnostic value in an infant or young child who has diarrhea; a negative assay, of course, indicates that C. difficile is not involved.

Antimicrobial-associated diarrhea not caused by C. difficile

C. difficile appears to be responsible for approximately

one-fourth to one-third of all cases of antimicrobial associated diarrhea. In the majority of the remainder of cases, evaluation fails to uncover a pathogen, although an enteric pathogen or S. aureus may be the cause of diarrhea in a small minority of cases. It has been recognized that antimicrobial therapy may upset the homeostasis of the normal bowel flora; this homeostasis or "colonization resistance" is thought to prevent proliferation of potential enteric pathogens that might gain access to the gut. Anecdotal reports suggest that the risk of development of diarrhea due to certain enteric pathogens, such as Salmonella, is increased by antimicrobial therapy. In addition, the possibility that antimicrobial therapy might be coincidental to the development of enteritis should be considered. Thus, in the patient who apparently has antimicrobial-associated diarrhea that does not involve C. difficile, it is appropriate to culture the feces for Campylobacter, Salmonella, Shigella, and Yersinia and to examine fecal smears for Entamoeba histolytica and Giardia.

Staphylococcus aureus was, at one time, considered to be the major cause of antimicrobial-associated diarrhea. Some investigators, however, have recently questioned whether or not S. aureus has any role in the development of antimicrobial-related diarrhea (Bartlett and Gorbach, 1977). Although retrospective analysis of published data is always fraught with difficulties, much of the older literature regarding S. aureus and antimicrobial-related diarrhea is more consistent with staphylococcal intestinal colonization than with staphylococcal-induced diarrhea. It is, in fact, quite reasonable to presume that many (but not all) of the putative cases of S. aureus enteritis were unrecognized cases of C. difficile-induced diarrhea. Although S. aureus produces a variety of toxins, none has convincingly been shown to be involved in antimicrobial-associated colitis. Since discovery of the role of C. difficile in the etiology of diarrhea, less than 15 cases of antimicrobial-associated S. aureus diarrhea have been reported (McDonald et al., 1982). Moreover, a mechanism by which S. aureus might cause diarrhea has not been demonstrated. Nonetheless, the feces should probably be cultured for S. aureus whenever neither C. difficile nor other bona fide enteric pathogens (vide supra) are detected in an apparent case of antimicrobial agent-associated diarrhea; a selective staphylococcal medium, such as mannitol salt agar should be adequate.

TREATMENT OF ANTIMICROBIAL AGENT-ASSOCIATED COLITIS OR DIARRHEA

General aspects of therapy

An essential aspect of therapy is the discontinuation of the antimicrobial agent that induced the diarrhea, in all but the most trivial cases of diarrhea. If continued therapy is indicated, then an agent that is equally effective, but unlikely to cause diarrhea should be given. In general, penicillins, cephalosporins, lincosamides (e.g., clindamycin) and macrolides (e.g., erythromycin) are relatively common causes of diarrhea whereas agents such as vancomycin, chloramphenicol, metronidazole and aminoglycosides (e.g., gentamicin) when administered parenterally, are unlikely to cause diarrhea. For example, it would be appropriate to change therapy of a gram-negative bacillary urinary tract infection from ampicillin to gentamicin if significant diarrhea were to develop during ampicillin treatment.

Adequate replacement of fluid and electrolyte losses is important, particularly in the debilitated, the very young and the elderly patient. It may be necessary on occasion to administer replacement fluids intravenously, particularly if nausea and vomiting are present.

Treatment of C. difficile-induced diarrhea

In addition to the above-mentioned general measures for treatment of antimicrobial-associated diarrhea, certain specific forms of therapy *may* be indicated whenever *C. difficile* is involved.

Use of antimicrobials active vs. C. difficile. Whenever *C. difficile* is thought to be the cause of diarrhea one must decide whether or not the diarrhea is severe enough to warrant therapy with an agent to rid the gut of this organism (George *et al*., 1980). Although vancomycin, metronidazole and bacitracin given orally all have been used to treat *C. difficile*-induced diarrhea, the greatest clinical experience by far is with vancomycin. Virtually all patients treated have responded to orally-administered vancomycin (Bartlett, 1983 ; Silva *et al*., 1981 ; Mogg *et al*, 1980 ; Keighley *et al* 1978a) usually within 24 to 48 hours of initiation of therapy. Vancomycin however, should not be given parenterally because this route of administration usually results in undetectable levels of drug in the large bowel contents; oral administration of 500 to 2,000 mg daily in four divided doses, on the other, produces fecal levels of drug that are several hundred-fold higher than the concentration needed to kill C. difficile (Keighley et al., 1978b; George et al., 1980 ; Tedesco et al., 1978a). The concentrations of vancomycin, metronidazole and bacitracin needed to kill C. difficile are all quite low (George et al., 1980); unfortunately, the information regarding fecal levels of metronidazole and bacitracin is too limited to permit the use of these agents in the patient with moderately severe to severe C. difficile-induced diarrhea.

Vancomycin (and metronidazole or bacitracin) should not be given to every patient with C. difficile-induced diarrhea because the disease is often self-limited (George et al., 1980) and because relapse of C. difficile diarrhea after completion of this type of therapy occurs in approximately 15 to 25% of patients treated (Bartlett et al., 1980a; Bartlett, 1983). In addition the use of vancomycin for treatment of a very mild case of diarrhea may not be warranted because of the high cost of the drug (George et al., 1980 ; Bartlett, 1983).

Metronidazole has generally been effective for treatment of C. difficile-induced diarrhea (George et al., 1980 ; Cherry et al., 1982; Brown, 1981 ; Nicolopoulos et al., 1981). The dose employed for adults has been 500 mg of metronidazole by mouth every 6 to 8 hours for 7 to 14 days. An appropriate dose for treatment of C. difficile-induced diarrhea in children has not been established; therefore it would be prudent not to use metronidazole for treatment of C. difficile-induced diarrhea in children except in unusual circumstances.

Similarly, orally-administered bacitracin (25,000 units four times daily for 7 to 10 days) has been effective for treatment of C. difficile-induced diarrhea in a few adult patients (Chang et al., 1980b; Tedesco, 1980). Because of the very limited experience with metronidazole and bacitracin, these agents should not be used in place of orally-administered vancomycin in patients who are severely ill except in the case of allergy to oral vancomycin or in countries in which vancomycin is not available (Bartlett, 1983).

Use of anionic exchange resins to bind C. difficile toxin. Cholestyramine and colestipol are anionic exchange resins that have been found to bind the cytotoxin of *C. difficile* *in vitro* and *in vivo* (George *et al*., 1980 ; Bartlett, 1983). Based on these data and earlier anecdotal experiences with cholestyramine for treatment of antimicrobial-associated pseudomembranous colitis (a disease that is now known to be due almost invariably to *C. difficile*), some investigators have recommended anionic exchange resins for treatment of *C. difficile*-induced diarrhea.

Colestipol, however, has been found to be no more effective than placebo in terms of producing a fall in *C. difficile* toxin titer in feces or clinical improvement in disease (Mogg *et al*., 1982). Although cholestyramine may provide benefit to some patients with *C. difficile*-associated diarrhea, it is vastly inferior to vancomycin (Bartlett, 1983). Well-designed controlled studies have not been done, but the available evidence suggests that cholestyramine *might* produce some benefit in approximately one half of patients with *C. difficile*-induced diarrhea (Keusch and Present, 1976 ; Bartlett, 1983). Cholestyramine, therefore should probably not be used (at least as the sole agent) for treatment of moderately severe to severe disease. Although cholestyramine will bind vancomycin to some extent (King and Barriere, 1981), the residual vancomycin appears to be adequate. Some investigators have suggested that optimal therapy would be orally administered vancomycin plus cholestyramine. Current data, however, indicate neither a benefit nor a detriment conferred by the addition of cholestyramine to vancomycin.

Specific recommendations for treatment of C. difficile-induced diarrhea. Guidelines for treatment of *C. difficile*-induced diarrhea can be summarized as follows (George *et al*., 1980 ; Bartlett, 1983):

1. For the mildly to moderately symptomatic patient: (a) discontinue the offending antimicrobial agent; this alone may be adequate; (b) consider administering cholestyramine in a dose of 4 grams every 6 hours; and (c) if diarrhea does not abate within 3 days, then discontinue cholestyramine and give vancomycin 0.125 grams by mouth 4 times daily for 7 to 10 days; metronidazole or bacitracin may be reasonable alternative (*vide supra*). The dose of vancomycin given to children is 500 mg/1.73 meter^2 by mouth every 6 hours (Batts *et*

al., 1980).

2. For the seriously ill patient: (a) discontinue the offending antimicrobial agent, if possible; and (b) begin vancomycin 0.5 grams by mouth every 6 hours for 7 to 14 days.

There are no data to support the use of other modalities of therapy such as antimicrobials (other than those mentioned above), Lactobacillus preparations, corticosteroids and antiperistaltic agents. Anecdotal experience suggests that antiperistaltic agents may predispose to development of toxic dilatation of the colon (George et al., 1980).

Management of relapse of C. difficile-induced diarrhea. Relapse of C. difficile colitis has been well-documented (George et al., 1979d, Bartlett et al., 1980a; Bartlett 1983 ; Chang et al., 1980b) . Patients who have had resolution of all symptoms of C. difficile-associated diarrhea during treatment with vancomycin (or, occasionally, bacitracin or metronidazole) may develop relapse of disease from several days to 5 or 6 weeks after discontinuation of vancomycin. It is important to realize that a significant proportion of patients with C. difficile-induced diarrhea will have resolution of symptoms as a consequence of discontinuation of the inciting agent. Prevention of relapse by avoiding indiscriminate use of vancomycin (or metronidazole and bacitracin) is an important aspect of management.

Relapse cannot be distinguished clinically from the original illness; it is associated with the presence of fecal cytotoxin, occurs in 15 to 25% of patients treated with oral vancomycin for C. difficile-associated diarrhea and may be recurrent (George et al., 1979d; Bartlett et al., 1980b). Vancomycin therapy invariably produces resolution of symptoms of relapse but clearly does not always prevent recurrence of relapse. A tapering dose schedule of vancomycin plus cholestipol has been found to be effective by one investigator (Tedesco, 1982a), whereas a standard course of vancomycin followed by a two to three week course of cholestyramine was found by another investigator to prevent recurrence of relapse (Bartlett, 1983); although the number of subjects treated with these two regimens is limited, the preliminary results are quite promising. The use of one of these regimens would represent the most reasonable approach available for management of relapse.

Special considerations. Although large bowel resection has been performed in the past for treatment of fulminating or intractable colitis, the efficacy of vancomycin should almost invariably obviate the need for resectional surgery (George *et al.*, 1980). Surgery may be required in some instances, however, because the development of ileus or toxic megacolon (both of which may occur in association with *C. difficile*-associated diarrhea) precludes the effective use of orally-administered vancomycin; parenteral administration of metronidazole, plus instillation of vancomycin directly into the bowel via ileostomy or colostomy, or both, is a potentially useful, but untested means of therapy in such cases (George *et al.*, 1980). Limited anecdotal experience suggests that the outcome of illness is quite poor when *C. difficile*-induced diarrhea is complicated by ileus or toxic dilatation of the colon (Cone and Wetzel, 1982).

Treatment of antimicrobial-associated diarrhea not caused by *C. difficile*.

As indicated above in the section on diagnosis, *C. difficile* is the cause of virtually all cases of antimicrobia-associated pseudomembranous colitis and approximately one-fourth of cases of antimicrobial-associated diarrhea in which a pseudomembrane is not found. Pseudomembranous colitis is, in general, a more severe disease than are the other types of antimicrobial-associated diarrhea. The occasional case of antimicrobial-associated diarrhea attributable to *S. aureus* should respond to treatment with oral vancomycin as outlined for *C. difficile* above. The infrequent cases of antimicrobial-associated diarrhea that appears to involve *Campylobacter*, *Salmonella*, *Shigella*, *Yersinia*, *Entamoeba* or *Giardia* should be treated the same as if antimicrobial therapy had not been a contributing factor; excellent reviews of these topics are available.

Guidelines for management of antimicrobial-associated diarrhea that does not involve a recognized pathogen have not been developed. Vancomycin has been shown not to be effective in such cases (Keighley *et al.*, 1978b); information regarding the efficacy of *Lactobacillus* preparations, corticosteroids, antiperistaltic agents and anionic exchange resins does not exist. Because this type of diarrhea tends to be mild, it may be most appropriate (and effective) simply to discontinue the offending antimicrobial.

SUMMARY

Antimicrobial-associated diarrhea is often caused by Clostridium difficile; this disease can best be diagnosed by detection of fecal cytotoxin in a tissue culture assay and, when therapy is indicated, can be effectively treated with orally administered vancomycin. The cause of disease in most cases of antimicrobial-associated diarrhea that do not involve C. difficile is not known; fortunately, this form of diarrhea is usually mild. Antimicrobial-associated diarrhea may also rarely involve S. aureus and certain enteric pathogens.

CHAPTER 4

DETECTION, ISOLATION AND IDENTIFICATION OF CLOSTRIDIUM DIFFICILE

S. P. BORRIELLO and PAULINE HONOUR

INDEX

DETECTION ISOLATION AND IDENTIFICATION OF CLOSTRIDIUM DIFFICILE

S.P. Borriello and Pauline Honour

Introduction

In view of the mounting evidence generated world wide in the last few years that firmly implicates *C. difficile* as the aetiological agent in both antibiotic and non-antibiotic associated pseudomembranous colitis (Larson *et al*., 1978, Bartlett *et al*., 1978a, George *et al*., 1978a), and also recent recognition of the fact that there may be a spectrum of gastrointestinal diseases associated with *C. difficile* infections (Borriello and Larson, 1981, Bolton *et al*., 1980, Brettle *et al*., 1982), an increasing number of laboratories are seeking to detect, isolate and identify *C. difficile* from clinical samples. The aims of this chapter are to critically review the methods currently available and to highlight problems that may arise.

Detection of *C. difficile* in stools

Direct methods

Direct microscopy for *C. difficile* using Gram stains of faecal smears, has not proved to be helpful in the detection of the organism; although Bartlett (1980) observed that when they examined Gram films of stools from patients with *C. difficile* colitis, some patients had clumps of Gram-positive cocci associated with white cells which would have satisfied diagnostic criteria used in cases of *Staphylococcus aureus* enterocolitis. Recently, McDonald *et al*., (1982) in describing an epidemic of hospital acquired infection due to *S. aureus* commented again on the distinctive Gram stained appearance of faecal smears in this condition. So, although direct microscopy of faecal smears may be of some benefit for the diagnosis of *S. aureus* associated enterocolitis there is no evidence to suggest it is useful for *C. difficile* associated diseases.

There have been a number of attempts to develop a method which would allow direct visualisation of *C. difficile* in clinical specimens by use of immunofluorescent (IF) techniques. Wilson *et al*., (1982b) evaluated a direct fluorescent-antibody (FA) test which was compared prospectively with orthodox laboratory isolation methods. They found that of 158 faecal specimens from patients with antibiotic-associated diarrhoea 30 were positive by the FA test (19%), and 32 by culture/toxin detection (20%). Although there was some discordance between the methods used with the FA test seemingly giving 6 false positive and 5 false negative results

(Table 1), detailed analysis of these cases led the authors to conclude that there was only one clealry false-positive result. However, 25 of 39 healthy adults were also positive by the FA test and only 4 of these 25 had C. difficile or cytotoxin present (Table 1). In addition, a positive FA test did not accurately predict the presence of C. difficile in subjects with diarrhoea unrelated to antibiotic therapy (Table 1). As the conjugate used in this study also reacted with some other species of clostridia ie. C. sordellii, C. bifermentans, C. chauvoei and C. sporogenes, it is possible that the false positive results noted in this study could have been due to cross-reactions with components of the faecal flora. Attempts to overcome this problem by improving the specificity of the conjugate by absorption with C. sordellii led to a loss of reactivity to other clostridia as well as to 18 of 20 isolates of C. difficile. This lack of specificity has also been noted by other workers (Lowe et al., 1980, see also section on identification).

Table 1

Fluorescent labelled antibody for the detection of Clostridium Difficile in stool specimens

Fluorescent labelled antibody	Clostridium difficile/toxin					
	Positive			Negative		
	A	B	C	A	B	C
Positive	26	3	4	5	7	21
Negative	6	1	1	121	8	13

Legend - A = antibiotic associated diarrhoea.
B = Diarrhoea unrelated to antibiotics
C = Healthy adults
Figure compiled from the data of Wilson et al 1982b.

A fluorescent labelled antibody has also been raised by Hubert et al., (1981) and shown to be effective for detecting C. difficile in the caecal contents of hamsters, and when used to estimate the number of bacteria present consistently gave higher values than those estimated by direct counts on a selective medium. Although these workers did not find cross-reactivity with a variety of different micro-organisms we found their conjugate cross-reacted with a strain of C. perfringens and C. sordellii.

Indirect methods

The indirect method most widely used as an indication of the presence or absence of C. difficile in clinical specimens is the demonstration of C. difficile cytotoxin in that specimen. There is a high degree of concordance between the presence or absence of this toxin and presence or absence of C. difficile (Borriello and Larson, 1981). The methods used for detection of this toxin are described in chapter 5 and will not therefore be dealt with here. The method relies on the ability of

C. difficile to produce cytotoxin in vivo. Recently Te-Wen Chang and Gorbach (1982) described an indirect method for detection of C. difficile by the in vitro production of cytotoxin in a selective enrichment broth. The technique involves the inoculation of an aliquot of faeces from a suspect patient into a chopped meat broth or onto blood agar medium incorporating cycloserine and cefoxitin as selective agents. Post incubation the broths, or agar plugs removed from the vicinity of suspect colonies on the agar medium, are analysed for the presence of cytotoxin. The advantage of this technique is that some stool samples that were negative for cytotoxin on initial screening were subsequently shown to have cytotoxigenic strains of C. difficile present capable of producing cytotoxin in vitro upon incubation in the selective medium. The authors maintain that their observations supported the concept that stool culture is more sensitive than stool toxin assay in making an aetiological diagnosis and propose the use of culture medium in addition to direct toxin detection in stools from patients with antibiotic-associated diarrhoea. The major problem with the broth enrichment method is that it would not permit the detection of non-cytotoxigenic strains. The authors maintain that they have not encountered toxin-negative C. difficile and further go on to propose that the difficulty of differentiating C. sporogenes from C. difficile may explain the controversial reports on the recovery of these non-toxigenic strains. This proposal, with respect to the statement made, needs discussion. The well documented reports of non-toxigenic C. difficile have come from laboratories with a long history of interest in C. difficile associated gastrointestinal disease and, more importantly, with laboratory personnel that have an expertise in clostridial identification. In addition, C. sporogenes does not grow on the selective medium employed for C. difficile isolation and, despite the contention of Te-Wen Chang and Gorbach, is not at all difficult to differentiate from C. difficile. The recent reports of the isolation of strains of C. difficile that only produced detectable levels of 'enterotoxin' as opposed to cytotoxin highlight the possible inadequacies of techniques that rely on detection of cytotoxin as an indication of the presence of C. difficile (Aronsson et al., 1982a).

Direct gas-liquid chromatography of stools has been proposed as a method for screening specimens for C. difficile. This method relies on the detection of isocaproic acid in faecal specimens (Potvliege et al., 1981). However, despite their belief that the technique seems a good screening method for excluding C. difficile infection, analysis of their data shows that they would have missed 39% of their C. difficile positive samples (Borriello, 1981b).

Isolation of C. difficile

The most common material submitted for the isolation of C. difficile is faecal specimens, although other clinical material such as ileostomy fluids, intestinal biopsies and blood cultures have been investigated for the presence of this organism. A variety of bacteriological methods to recover C. difficile from such material have been employed.

The first isolation of C. difficile, the organism then named as Bacillus difficilis, was reported in 1935 by Hall and O'Toole from their work on the faecal flora of breast-fed infants. They used a non-selective agar, indeed, until relatively recently, there were no selective media available. The first attempt to develop a selective isolation procedure developed from the observations of Elsden (1976), who showed that *C. difficile* produced *p*-cresol as a product of the metabolism of L-tyrosine, and that it was almost unique amongst the clostridia in this ability. This observation was utilized by Hafiz and Oakley (1976) who, working on the premise that if an organism produced *p*-cresol it must be resistant to the antimicrobial activity of that product, incorporated 0.2% (wt/vol) *p*-cresol into reinforced clostridial medium (RCM) to produce a selective enrichment broth. The major problem with any enrichment technique is that it can only be used to provide qualitative and not quantitative, data. An additional problem is that this selective broth is not specific for *C. difficile*. This is not surprising, especially as it has been shown that other clostridia can produce *p*-cresol from L-tyrosine and are presumably resistant to this metabolite (Bone *et al*., 1976). Other clostridial species such as *C. paraputrificum* as well as members of other genera, such as streptococci, have been recovered from this selective broth (Borriello, unpublished observations). Therefore, presence or absence of growth *per se*, including the so-called typical 'cornfield appearance', cannot be taken as indicative of the presence or absence of *C. difficile*. All enrichment broths showing growth should be sub-cultured onto an appropriate agar medium and the plates then screened post-incubation for colonies typical of *C. difficile*. Willey & Bartlett (1979) using this medium for the isolation of *C. difficile* from faeces in comparison with direct plating on to a selective agar, found that it was less sensitive and no more selective. Various workers have incorporated *p*-cresol into agar medium (George *et al*., 1979c), however it is the common experience that 0.2% of this agent is too inhibitory to be used as a selective additive to solid media and that when the concentration is reduced the selectivity of the media is lost. Recent methods for isolation have been greatly facilitated by the development of selective media (George *et al*., 1979c, Willey and Bartlett, 1979). George *et al*., recommended 500 µg/ml of cycloserine and 16 µg/ml of cefoxitin as selective agents in an egg yolk, fructose agar base (CCFA) whilst Willey and Bartlett reduced the cycloserine to 250 µg/ml and cefoxitin to 10 µg/ml and incoporated both into brain-heart infusion agar base with added 5% sheep blood. There are commercially available selective media based on these findings (Oxoid and Difco) both using 500 µg/ml of cycloserine, 16 µg/ml of cefoxitin and 7% horse blood. The procedure employed is simply to seed the selective agar plates with the sample to be analysed, either undiluted and/or diluted with an appropriate diluent such as brain-heart infusion broth. The plates are incubated in an anaerobic atmosphere of 80% Nitrogen, 10% Hydrogen and 10% carbon dioxide at 37°C for 24 to 48 hours. The plates are then screened for presumptive *C. difficile* colonies.

The colour of the colonies on the selective agar plates differs depending whether a blood or egg base is used, but on both, the colonial morphology is similar. They have a ground-glass appearance, 3-5 mm diameter, flat and irregular, with an undulate edge. Some strains produce white colonies. Recognition of colonies of *C. difficile* is greatly facilitated by viewing under long-wave (366 nm) ultra-violet light (George *et al.*, 1979c) as colonies of *C. difficile* exhibit a characteristic yellow green/chartreuse fluorescence. A green fluorescence is also evident on blood agar media (George *et al.*, 1979c, Borriello and Honour, 1981). Clostridia other than *C. difficile*, as well as other components of the faecal flora will grow on this selective medium and confusion can sometimes occur when other 'green' fluorescning colonies are encountered. However, our experience has been that when the colonies are examined in normal day-light they appear as flat, very green colonies whereas *C. difficile* appears as a greyish, 'ground-glass' colony. These organisms can be further distinguished from *C. difficile* by comparison of their respective gas-liquid chromatographic profiles of the volatile fatty acid end products of metabolism. To date the only colonies that could have caused confusion have been identified as *C. inocuum*, an organism that produces only acetic and butyric acid as volatile fatty acids. A less easy method for helping to recognise colonies of *C. difficile* is to remove agar plugs from the vicinity of the colony and to look for cytotoxin (see above) or to analyse the agar plugs for the presence of *p*-cresol (Phillips and Rogers 1981), a method which is more fully described in the section on identification.

One note of caution in using this selective agar is that some workers find that isolated colonies of *C. difficile* appear to be extremely oxygen sensitive and therefore should be sub-cultured into a suitable broth or re-plated onto a non-selective agar without delay.

Holst *et al.*, (1981) in Sweden have compared the use of cooked meat glucose broth with added cycloserine (500 μg/ml) and cefoxitin (10 μg/ml) to the selective agar described by George *et al.*, (1979c) when culturing stool samples from children. They found no difference in the recovery rate of *C. difficile* between the enrichment broth or plate method used.

Table 2

Procedures for the selective isolation of *Clostridium difficile*

Selective procedure	Reference
Broth enrichment with 0.2% *p*-cresol	Hafiz and Oakley, 1976.
Selection of spores by:	
(a) heat	Dowell and Hawkins 1974, Larson *et al.*, 1978.
(b) alcohol	Koransky *et al.*, 1978, Borriello and Honour, 1981.
Antibiotic containing selective media	George *et al.*, 1979c, Willey and Bartlett, 1979, Hubert *et al.*, 1981.

In addition to the selective media containing cycloserine and cefoxitin Hubert et al., (1981) described a minimal and selective medium containing five amino acids, three vitamins, a low sugar concentration and the incorporation of cefoxitin (16 μg/ml) and streptomycin (500 μg/ml) as selective agents. As far as we are aware this medium has not received widespread approval, probably due to the acceptance of the cycloserine-cefoxitin containing media, and the extra difficulty involved in the preparation of a minimal medium.

Spore selection techniques can be used either as an alternative to a selective medium or as a preliminary selection step before plating onto any medium. Heat treatment can be used to detect for spores at the expense of vegetative cells. The normal procedure is to expose dilutions of the material in question to 75°C for 20 minutes or 80°C for 10 minutes prior to plating on agar media (Dowell and Hawkins 1974, Borriello et al., 1978). We used heat treatment in our early work in addition to p-cresol enrichment broths for the selection of C. difficile (Larson et al., 1978, Borriello, 1979). A more sensitive method for the selection of clostridial spores is the use of ethanol (Koransky et al., 1978). In this method an aliquot of a low dilution of the material to be examined is mixed with an equal volume of absolute ethanol and left at room temperature for one hour before any further diluting and plating onto agar media. This method has been fully evaluated by Borriello and Honour (1981) and shown to be a very effective way of isolating C. difficile. Of 266 faecal samples analysed 82 were shown to be positive for C. difficile by a combination of the use of a cycloserine-cefoxitin selective agar (CCA) and alcohol spore selection. Of these 82 positive specimens, 77(94%) were detected by CCA and 72 (88%) by the alcohol spore selection procedure. Ten samples (12%) yielded C. difficile on CCA only, and five specimens (6%) only by the alcohol procedure. In most cases quantitative recovery was greater on the selective agar.

Both of these spore selection techniques use the ability of clostridial species to form endospores. The formation and germation of a bacterial spore is complex and can be affected by various manipulations. Ionesco (1978) has shown that spore germination maybe initiated by lysozyme and that treatment of the spores with the reducing agent sodium thioglycollate in the presence of lysozyme at a concentration of 5 μg/ml allows for the germination of 'superdormant' spores. The results of this study show that the addition of lysozyme will result in a 10^3-fold greater recovery and that a combination of pre-treatment with sodium thioglycollate and lysozyme results in a 10^5-fold increase in recovery of C. difficile. The implications of these findings in situations where small numbers of organisms are being looked for are obvious. Nakamura et al., (1981a) also used lysozyme (10 μg/ml) added to selective media to increase the germination of spores of C. difficile.

Raibaud and co-workers (1974) have shown that they can augment the outgrowth of clostridial spores from faecal specimens by the addition to the media of 1% sodium taurocholate and further that recovery of C. difficile is enhanced on such media (Raibaud et al., 1980). We have routinely incorporated sodium taurocholate into our selective medium since 1979 (based on a presentation by Raibaud) and found this procedure improves our recovery of C. difficile. In addition we have noted that although the incorporation of sodium taurocholate into our medium resulted in higher yields of C. difficile when working with isolates, the further addition of lysozyme to this medium did not further improve recovery. However, there was some improvement in the quantitative recovery of C. difficile from stools, when using the lysozyme containing medium (unpublished observations). The use of sodium taurocholate was more fully evaluated by Wilson et al., (1982a), who showed that media incorporating sodium taurocholate was more sensitive for detecting C. difficile in patient specimens, and usually yielded a heavier growth of the organism than the routine selective medium.

Environmental 'sampling' has been simplified by the use of contact plates (Nunc-Gibco) containing cycloserine-cefoxitin selective agar which can be used to sample from 100-500 cm^2 of suspect surface area. In some places, where contact plates are not convenient, a swab pre-moistened with 0.85% NaCl can be used to sample and then inoculate plate or broth media.

In general, recovery of C. difficile from surfaces in the environment eg. walls and floors of hospital wards has been poor. It is possible that this is a reflection of the insensitivity of the methods used. If one accepts that these environments are inhospitable to C. difficile then they probably exist there as superdormant spores requiring activation before they will germinate. Working on this premise we have shown in 'seeding experiments' that contact plates containing a selective media incorporating lysozyme are superior to those that do not, for the recovery of C. difficile from the surface of a tile 8 days after it has been 'seeded' and left exposed at room temperature in air (unpublished observations).

Although the addition of lysozyme to media had no signficiant effect when looking at the recovery of C. difficile from patients with antibiotic-associated diarrhoea, or laboratory isolates, this is probably due to the relatively small numbers of C. difficile spores that require activation by lysozyme that are present, so that even if these spores do germinate the effect on total recovery would be negligible. However, when looking at material where very small numbers may be present such as the stools of healthy people, or exposed inanimate hospital ward surfaces, both of which are probably inhospitable environments, then one may expect the relative number of activation requiring superdormant spores to be much higher. An optimum method for the recovery of C. difficile from the environment may be to place used swabs into sodium thioglycolate and to then transfer them to an enrichment medium containing both sodium taurocholate and lysozyme.

Identification of C. difficile

As with most other newly encountered organisms, recognition of C. difficile becomes easier with experience; in particular, its distinctive 'horsey' odour is helpful in recognition. On blood agar plates incubated anaerobically at 37°C for 48 to 72 h, C. difficile appears as irregular, convex colonies 3-5 mm in diameter often with a whitish, matt, rough surface but sometimes the colonies are flat greyish and appear to have a 'greenish' tinge in the media around their edge. The cellular morphology of C. difficile after 48 to 72 h incubation on a non-selective blood agar plate, as seen by Gram film can be characteristic Gram-positive rods (4.8 μm x 0.5 - 1 μm) with subterminal to terminal oval spores which sometimes occur at both ends of the rod to give a 'dumb-bell' appearance (Borriello and Honour, 1981).

Methods that are commonly used for further identification of *C. difficile* are gas-liquid chromatography (GLC) and biochemical reaction profiles. *C. difficile* produces the following short chain fatty acids, acetic, proprionic, iso-butyric, butyric, iso-valeric, valeric, iso-caproic, lactic and succinic and small amounts of caproic as end products of metabolism in a chopped meat carbohydrate broth. These compounds are readily detected by GLC techniques (Holdeman *et al.*, 1977). Identification of the fatty acids produced is based upon comparison of their relative retention times compared to those of known standards. It is important that adequate reference standards or an extract of an organism such as *C. sporogenes* which produces variable amounts of a range of volatile fatty acids (VFA) should be used as controls. Although the VFA profile is characteristic there is a report that asaccharolytic strains of *C. difficile* fail to produce valeric acid (Poxton 1982), however we have never encountered strains that were unable to do this. From a qualitative point of view *C. difficile* and *C.* sporogenes give similar volatile fatty acid profiles, but the yield of these fatty acids is far greater from *C. sporogenes*.

The increased resolution and separating capacity of silica-glass capillary columns has been applied to the detection of a variety of metabolic end products of *C. difficile* (Wayne-Moss and Nunez-Montiel 1982), however, the complexity of the derivatisation and extraction procedures would limit its usefulness for most routine laboratories.

As previously mentioned Elsden *et al.*, have shown that *C. difficile* produces *p*-cresol as an end point of tyrosine metabolism, and noted that *p*-hydroxyphenyl acetic acid (HPA) was a precursor. On the basis of this observation Phillips & Rogers (1981) have used a GLC technique to demonstrate the presence of *p*-cresol produced from HPA incorporated into the agar medium by the removal and analysis of agar plugs taken from culture plates of pure cultures of *C. difficile* and/or cultures of stools containing *C. difficile*. They admit that the distinctive odour of *p*-cresol which was often discernible on examination of culture plates made the GLC findings essentially confirmatory. Our reservation of this technique is that insufficient work has been done to determine how many other species of bacteria can produce *p*-cresol from HPA. It is worth noting that blood base agar media contain sufficient levels of tyrosine for the production of detectable levels of *p*-cresol by *C. difficile*.

Nunez-Montiel *et al.*, (1983) have recently described a new medium, norleucine-tyrosine broth which is a trypticase, yeast-extract-salts base with added 0.2% (wt/vol) L-norleucine and 0.2% (wt/vol) L-tyrosine which they use for identification of cultures of *C. difficile* on the basis of caproic acid and *p*-cresol production. Using normal ether extraction procedures on a 48 hour norleucine-tyrosine broth culture, all strains of *C. difficile* tested by GLC produced both caproic acid and *p*-cresol whereas no other micro-organism tested were found to produce both of these products in this broth.

In most cases attempts to produce different growth media to alter the types of metabolic end-products readily detected by GLC are based on the assumption that *C. difficile* and *C. sporogenes* produce the same volatile fatty acid profile and are therefore difficult to differentiate. These assumptions are incorrect, as the two organisms are readily differentiated on a variety of simple tests (Table 3).

Table 3

Differentiation of *Clostridium difficile* and *Clostridium sporogenes*

Test	C. difficile	C. sporogenes
Growth on selective medium	+	-
Fluorescence under long-wave ultra-violet light	+	-
Rapid digestion of meat	-	+
Characteristic smell	'horsey'	foul, putrefactive
Production of *p*-cresol from L-tyrosine	+	-

As for most other anaerobes, confirmation of identity is based on the results of a range of biochemical reaction tests. Optimally, these are performed by using the methods described by Holdeman *et al*., (1977). However the situation in many routine laboratories is that the same type of media that is generally used for aerobes is employed, which is obviously less satisfactory. In order to overcome the problems of lack of suitable media many laboratories now use commercially available test systems that are specifically designed for anaerobes. In our experience interpretation of weak reactions by *C. difficile* in the API 20A system, which is the most commonly used commercial system, can prove to be difficult. In addition, whichever method of obtaining biochemical reaction profiles is used, it has been our experience, shared with others (Poxton 1982), that there is a fair degree of strain variability which complicates attempts to identify the organism. Because of these problems the majority of laboratories rely on combinations of colonial and cellular morphology, fluorescence under long-wave ultra-violet light, growth on selective media, cytotoxin production and detection of the characteristic fatty acid end products of metabolism.

More recently immuno-techniques have been used for identification of *C. difficile*. The use of fluorescent labelled antibody and enzyme immuno-assays for the detection of *C. difficile* in faecal specimens have already been described. These techniques could also be applied to the rapid presumptive identification of suspect colonies of *C. difficile*. The majority of immuno-techniques used for the identification of *C. difficile* are based on the detection of *C. difficile* cytotoxin (Welch *et al*., 1980), or at least thought to be based on cytotoxin detection, and are dealt with in chapter 5.

Polyacrylamide gel electrophoresis has been used for the analysis of soluble proteins and has been investigated as a method for identifying clostridia, including *C. difficile* (Cato *et al.*, 1982). Finally, the observation of Barclay and Borriello (1982) that certain strains of *C. beijerinckii* inhibit the growth of *C. difficile* but have no comparable effect against any other organism tested led to the suggestion that sensitivity to *C. beijerinckii* may be useful as a rapid method for the presumptive identification of *C. difficile* isolates.

CHAPTER 5

DETECTION OF CLOSTRIDIUM DIFFICILE TOXINS

S. P. BORRIELLO and A. R. WELCH

INDEX

DETECTION OF CLOSTRIDIUM DIFFICILE TOXINS

S.P. Borriello and A.R. Welch

Introduction

C. difficile has been shown to account for up to 47% of antibiotic associated diarrhoea (Borriello and Larson 1981). Laboratory diagnosis of C. difficile in human faecal specimens has used selective culture media and the detection of cytotoxin (toxin B).

Until recently, the cytotoxicity assay was the only procedure available for the routine detection of cytotoxin which has restricted this test to laboratories with access to tissue culture facilities. Because of this there has been much interest in the development of physio-chemical methods to replace cytotoxicity assays. In this chapter these tests, as well as the standard cytotoxicity assay for detection of C. difficile toxin, will be discussed.

Detection of C. difficile cytotoxin (Toxin B)

There are a number of methods currently available for the detection and quantitation of C. difficile cytotoxin. The most widely employed method is the use of tissue culture.

Tissue culture

Detection of C. difficile cytotoxin using tissue culture methods is a simple rapid and sensitive aid in the diagnosis of C. difficile infections. Chang et al., (1979[a]) and more recently Donta et al., (1982) and Guigliano et al., (1982) have assessed the sensitivities of a variety of mammalian cell lines (Table 1).

In our laboratory we routinely use monolayers of Vero cells grown in tubes. The growth medium consists of medium 199 with 5% (vol/vol) foetal calf serum (Flow laboratories). Once confluent the cells are maintained in the same medium with 1% (vol/vol) foetal calf serum. Both growth and maintenance media contain penicillin and streptomycin at final concentrations of 100 units and 100 µg per ml respectively.

The advantage in using Vero cells is that they are a continuous cell line and undergo rapid cell multiplication, an important factor if a large number of specimens are to be routinely tested for the presence of cytotoxin

Although we use tissue culture treated glass test tubes for preparation of monolayers, many workers use plastic tubes, and microtitre plates which are especially useful for screening larger numbers of specimens (Borriello

Table 1

Cell Line tested

Primary human amnion[1]	African green monkey kidney (Vero)[2]
Baby hamster kidney (BHK21)[1]	Adult rhesus monkey kidney (LLC-MK2)
HeLa	Rat hepatoma (MHC)
Human diploid lung fibroblasts (Wl-38)	Dog kidney epithelial cells (MDCK)
Rabbit kidney (RK)	Embryonic human intestine (INT-407)
Rabbit kidney (RK-13)	Human embryonic foreskin (HFS)[2]
Chinese hamster ovary (CHO-K1)	Human embryonic lung (MRC-5)[1]
Mouse areolar and adipose tissue (L929)[1,2]	Mouse adrenal tumours (YI)[3]

Legend
1. Shown to be most sensitive by Chang *et al*., (1979[a])
2. Shown to be most sensitive by Guigliano *et al*., (1982)
3. Shown to be most sensitive by Donta *et al*., (1982).

1978, George, 1979). The procedure used for *C. difficile* cytotoxin detection in stool specimens in our laboratory is as follows.

An approximate 1:10 suspension of stool in Hanks Balanced Salt solution (Hanks BSS) is prepared, thoroughly mixed and centrifuged at 12,000 rpm for 30 minutes at 4°C. The supernatant is then carefully removed using a Pasteur pipette, if the supernatant appears cloudy it is filtered through a disposable 0.45 μ filter.

A 0.1 ml aliquot of the supernatant is then added to a Vero cell monolayer. Cytotoxicity is recorded after overnight incubation on a roller drum at 37°C. The cytopathic effect (CPE) is distinctive and the presence of *C. difficile* cytotoxin can be confirmed by neutralisation with the cross reacting *C. sordellii* antitoxin, which is available from Wellcome Research Laboratories, and is used at the recommended dilution of 1:50 in PBSA. Normal horse serum, also at a dilution of 1:50, is used as a control for non-specific neutralisation by the horse raised antiserum. Once prepared the antitoxin is stable for a number of weeks at 4°C.

The following neutralisation procedure is recommended (Fig. 1).

Figure 1.

	Test	Control
Specimen	0.1 ml stool supernatant + 0.1 ml *C. sordellii* antitoxin.	0.1 ml stool supernatant + 0.1 ml normal horse serum.
C. difficile Control.	0.1 ml *C. difficile* culture filtrate + 0.1 ml *C. sordellii* antitoxin	0.1 ml toxigenic *C. difficile* culture filtrate + 0.1 ml normal horse serum.

The tubes are then incubated overnight at 37°C. If the CPE is due to C. difficile cytotoxin, no CPE should be present in tubes containing stool supernatant mixed with C. sordellii antitoxin. However, the CPE should be present in tubes containing stool supernatant mixed with normal horse serum.

The major limitation on this type of toxin detection system is the acceptance that sophisticated facilities and expertise are required for tissue culture techniques. However we have shown that most of these limitations can be readily overcome. The maintenance of a stock of Vero cells is relatively simple and could be carried out in a routine microbiology laboratory. The lack of an inverted microscope and specific tissue culture tubes can be overcome by simply growing the Vero cells on glass cover-slips. The cover-slip monolayers of Vero cells can be transferred to a petri dish containing maintenance medium and challenged with the sample to be tested, e.g. faecal filtrate, incubated at 37°C in a CO_2 incubator and viewed by conventional light microscopy under low magnification. The cells can be readily stained by crystal violet to facilitate screening. A simple alternative to glass cover-slips is the 8 chamber, tissue culture slide now available commercially (Miles Scientific). We have recently successfully introduced both methods in a pilot study into a routine microbiology laboratory.

Enzyme-immunoassays

Enzyme linked immunosorbent assays (ELISA) have been developed for the two C. difficile toxins so far described.

Yolken et al., (1981) have developed an indirect ELISA for detection of the cytotoxin (Toxin B) in patient stool specimens. Using microtitre plates coated with rabbit C. difficile antiserum, stool supernatants prepared in PBS at pH 7.2 were added and the presence of toxin B detected by incubation with C. difficile antiserum raised in goats, and subsequent incubations with anti-goat IgG alkaline phosphatase conjugate and p-nitrophenol phosphate substrate. The plates were then read either by eye or by using a microplate colorimeter. These workers found minimal reactivity with isolated strains of C. bifermentans and C. sporogenes but not with 15 other species of clostridia nor 45 strains of aerobic bacteria. However, their system also detected strains of toxigenic C. sordellii which produce an immunologically similar toxin (unpublished).

A comparison of ELISA and cytotoxicity assay for detection of C. difficile toxin in stool specimens is presented in Table 2.

Table 2

Comparison of ELISA and tissue culture for the detection of C. difficile cytotoxin in faecal material

Tissue Culture	ELISA		
	Positive	Negative	Total
Positive	84	0	84
Negative	3*	190	193
Total	87	190	277

*2 of the 3 discrepant results were culture positive for C. difficile and the third was positive by cytotoxicity but had become negative following vancomycin treatment.

The use of ELISA for detection of C. difficile toxin is of value in that the enzyme immunoassay offers quantitative measurement of toxin levels in faecal specimens, it only requires small quantities of reagents, and most importantly allows laboratories without access to tissue culture facilities an opportunity to provide a rapid, sensitive and specific diagnostic test.

However, the ability for large numbers of specimens to be processed may not be of great value to many laboratories and we feel that it offers more to studies involving the epidemiology of C. difficile in human infection.

Counterimmunoelectrophoresis

The development of counterimmunoelectrophoresis (CIE) for detection of C.difficile cytotoxin has been attempted by a number of workers (Table 3). Welch et al., (1980) and Ryan et al., (1980) have developed CIE for detection of C. difficile cytotoxin in toxin containing culture filtrates and human faecal specimens respectively. However, doubt has been cast over the interpretation of their results by a number of workers. Poxton and Byrne (1981[a,b]) believe the antigen detected by these workers may not be C. difficile toxin but a cell surface antigen of C. difficile. They have demonstrated that C. difficile, C. sordellii and C. bifermentans have at least one surface carbohydrate antigen in common. This may account for strains of C. sordellii and C. bifermentans that are negative by cytotoxicity testing being positive by CIE (Welch et al., 1980) and why all C. difficile strains tested are positive by CIE although some are non-cytotoxigenic in tissue culture (Welch et al., 1980). West and Wilkins (1982) support the view that the precipitin bands obtained are probably due to C. difficile antigens other than cytotoxin. They have found that their C. difficile antitoxin will produce intense CIE reactions with strains of C. difficile that are known to be non-cytotoxigenic.

Table 3

Comparison of tissue culture and counterimmunoelectrophoresis for the detection of C. difficile cytotoxin in stools

Tissue Culture	Counterimmunoelectrophoresis	
	Positive	Negative
Positive	45	51
Negative	105	641

Legend

Figures compiled from Ryan et al., (1980), Levine et al., (1982), Wu and Fung (1983), Jarvis et al., (1983), Kurzynski et al., (1983), Sands et al., (1983).

The interest shown in the use of CIE as a diagnostic procedure for detection of C. difficile cytotoxin is due mainly to the lack of tissue culture facilities in many laboratories. It is potentially a fast sensitive procedure for use in a routine laboratory. However, the literature so far would suggest that although it is possible to detect C. difficile antigens, its use for detection of cytotoxin will be hampered until a purified specific antitoxin can be raised. This situation is exemplified in Table 3 where it can be seen that, if accepting tissue culture cytotoxicity as the standard against which to compare CIE, of 842 samples analysed 96 were positive by tissue culture and of these 96 CIE failed to detect toxin in 51. In addition CIE was positive for 105 'negative' samples. However, it is encouraging that of the 842 samples 641 were negative by both methods.

Detection of C. difficile enterotoxin (Toxin A)

Clostridium difficile has been shown to produce at least two toxins. One toxin produces a positive fluid response in rabbit ileal loops and has been designated C. difficile 'enterotoxin' (Toxin A). The other toxin is negative in the rabbit ileal loop and has been designated C. difficile cytotoxin (Toxin B).

This section will describe methods for the detection of C. difficile 'enterotoxin'.

Tissue culture

Both toxin A and toxin B of C. difficile are cytotoxic to a variety of different cell lines (Donta et al., 1982). However, toxin B (cytotoxin) is at least 1,000 times as active as toxin A (Sullivan et al., 1982). In general, unless one is looking at purified toxin preparations and/or has specific antitoxins available there is little to commend tissue culture as a system for the detection of toxin B, especially as it has been shown that using one of the most sensitive cell lines for this assay (Y1 cells) it was not possible to detect toxin A in toxin-containing stools of asymptomatic neonates or symptomatic adults (Donta et al., 1982).

Enzyme-immunoassays

Lyerly et al., (1983) have developed an enzyme-linked immunosorbent assay (ELISA) for the detection of toxin A in human faecal samples. Although the toxin A ELISA at present is not as sensitive as the cytotoxicity test for toxin B, work is currently being undertaken to increase the sensitivity of these techniques and will ultimately lead to further evaluation of toxin A in disease.

ANIMAL TEST SYSTEMS

Vascular Permeability

This procedure involves the intradermal injection of toxin preparations into the shaved backs of rabbits, the diameters of the skin reactions being measured at 6 hours and 18 hours. Vascular permeability is determined by intravenous injection of Evans blue dye at 18 hours post intradermal injection. Bluing diameters are then measured 3 hours later. As with the rabbit ileal loop assay, cholera toxin is used as a positive control. Using this technique Lyerly et al., (1982) found that 1 ng or greater of both toxin A and toxin B produced erythematous and/or haemorrhagic lesions, and at 10 ng or greater would cause an increase in vascular permeability. Overall, toxin A gave significantly greater lesions and bluing responses than toxin B.

Rabbit ileal loop

Ligated intestinal loops 5-7 cm in length are prepared and injected with 1 ml samples of toxin preparation. Cholera toxin is used to act as a positive control. After 10 hours the rabbits are sacrificed and a ratio of volume to length (ml per cm) determined for each loop. Lyerly et al., (1982) found using ligated rabbit loops that toxin A caused a viscous haemorrhagic fluid response, whereas toxin B produced only a weak variable fluid response, with no apparent haemorrhage.

Suckling mouse assay

Infant mice are inoculated intragastrically with toxin preparations and then anally occluded with cyanoacrylate ester glue. Four hours post infection the mice are sacrificed by cervical dislocation and the fluid accumulation ratio determined for each mouse. Lyerly et al., (1982) found that 0.5 μg doses or greater of toxin A (enterotoxin) caused a significant accumulation of fluid, whereas toxin B (cytotoxin) required 2.5 μg doses or greater to produce a significant response.

Mouse lethality

In a study of the biological activities of purified toxic fractions of spent culture medium from C. difficile Banno et al., (1981) showed that the fraction that was cytotoxin and failed to induce fluid accumulation in the rabbit ligated loop assay was also non lethal to mice upon intraperitoneal injection. However, the non-cytotoxic fraction was positive for both fluid accumulation and mouse lethality. These results imply that mouse lethality could be used as a method for detection of toxin A. In this respect it is of interest that we have some strains of C. difficile that are positive in the mouse lethality test but non-pathogenic to hamsters and non-cytotoxigenic in tissue culture (Borriello and Barclay, unpublished observations).

The use of animal models for demonstration of C. difficile toxin A are restricted mainly to research establishments. Because of variability in experimental results obtained using animals which may be dependent largely on personal expertise and recognising the need to reduce the use of animal models we feel that the development of physiochemical procedures such as ELISA should be actively encouraged.

SUMMARY

The detection of C. difficile cytotoxin (toxin B) has relied largely on the cytotoxicity test and neutralisation of the cytopathic effect observed by the cross-reacting C. sordellii antitoxin. Because of the lack of tissue culture facilities in many laboratories alternative physiochemical methods have been developed.

Countercurrent immunoelectrophoresis is a procedure widely used in many diagnostic microbiology laboratories and its use in detection of C.difficile cytotoxin looked promising in first reports. Its major advantage was that it was a quick, technically simple and inexpensive test. However, it has been shown that the antisera used in its evaluation proved to be too crude and detected other C. difficile antigens along with cytotoxin. It still has a role to play in indicating the presence of C. difficile in human faecal specimens, and when a commercial monospecific antiserum to C. difficile cytotoxin can be raised it would be a useful test for many laboratories. The use of animals to detect C. difficile enterotoxin (toxin A) are not useful to a diagnostic laboratory and are restricted to research establishments. However, the development of an ELISA technique for detection of C. difficile enterotoxin will be useful in determining its role in the course of human disease. The use of ELISA for detection of C. difficile cytotoxin however is not we feel of great value in a routine setting. The major advantage of the technique is that large numbers of faecal specimens can be tested, but in most routine diagnostic microbiology laboratories the number of specimens would be relatively small and the screening of all faecal specimens cannot be justified. At the present time the detection of C. difficile in faecal specimens is still dependent on isolation on selective media and demonstration of cytotoxin by cytotoxicity assay. We feel that the use of cytotoxicity assays could be performed in routine microbiology laboratories using the simplified tissue culture approach outlined above, and that attempts to develop simplified handling, maintenance and use of tissue cultures would be of benefit to a great number of laboratories.

CHAPTER 6

EPIDEMIOLOGY OF ANTIMICROBIAL AGENT-ASSOCIATED DIARRHOEA AND COLITIS

M. E. MULLIGAN

INDEX

EPIDEMIOLOGY OF ANTIMICROBIAL AGENT-ASSOCIATED DIARRHEA AND COLITIS

M.E. MULLIGAN

INTRODUCTION

The epidemiology of Clostridium difficile-induced intestinal disease is an important and intriguing subject not only because the disease is in many ways unique, but also because there are so many basic questions that remain to be answered. C. difficile appears to be a rather special pathogen: rarely harmful to the completely healthy host, but not known to be more pathogenic in the severely immunocompromised. Instead, most cases of C. difficile-induced diarrhea and colitis occur simply in association with antimicrobial therapy (Bartlett, 1979 ; Mogg et al., 1979); it appears that this alone is enough to alter host resistance to this organism. Indeed, altered intestinal ecology is one apparent risk factor for disease (Fekety et al., 1980); however the nature of this predisposing alteration is not yet fully understood. In addition, although the disease is frequently seen in seriously ill, elderly, hospitalized patients (Bartlett, 1979 ; Lusk et al., 1977 ; Mogg et al., 1979), the specific risk factors for this and other populations and the details of host defense are not yet identified. Furthermore, it has become apparent that there must be important unknown factors which, in addition to antimicrobial therapy and the presence of the organism, contribute to the development of the illness.

At present, it is not known whether disease is usually due to overgrowth of an organism that is part of the "normal flora" of some persons or instead a consequence of exposure to an external source of the pathogen at a time of susceptibility. C. difficile has been recovered from a wide variety of sources, but the epidemiological importance of these potential reservoirs is not yet defined. Interestingly, C. difficile-induced disease is commonly reported from some geographic areas (Tedesco et al., 1974a) but rarely recognized in others. Even within an institution, there appears to be variation in the frequency of the illness (Swartzberg et al., 1977). Despite remarkable advances in understanding the recently recognized pathogen, C. difficile, and its role in human disease, there are still many answered questions about the epidemiology.

SPECTRUM OF DISEASE

Before considering what is known about the epidemiology of C. difficile-induced diarrhea and colitis, it is wise to recall the spectrum of disease that can be attributed to this pathogen. C. difficile can be implicated in greater than 90% of cases of documented pseudomembranous colitis following antimicrobial therapy (Bartlett et al., 1980a; George et al., 1982). However, it appears that there may be other forms of colitis associated with antimicrobial agents. Several groups of workers, have described an apparently distinctive hemorrhagic colitis following treatment with various penicillins and related agents which may not be linked to C. difficile (Toffler, 1978 ; Sakurai et al., 1979 ; Hickling and Fuller, 1979). Furthermore, there is evidence for C. difficile as a pathogen in only an approximate 20 to 25% of cases of antibiotic-associated diarrhea (in which pseudomembranes are not demonstrated), suggesting that some other microorganism or some non-infectious etiology must be responsible for most of these cases (Bartlett et al., 1980a; Viscidi et al., 1981). Thus, the full details of the epidemiology of all antimicrobial agent-associated intestinal disease await elucidation of the etiology of cases not involving C. difficile. In addition, C. difficile-induced intestinal disease does not occur only in the setting of preceding antimicrobial therapy but also is reported, although uncommonly, in association with diverse other conditions (Fainstein et al., 1981 ; Thomas et al., 1982), and occasionally with no apparent underlying process (Peikin et al., 1980). Finally, it must be remembered that C. difficile may be present in the gastrointestinal tracts of persons receiving antimicrobial therapy who have no apparent resultant disease (Viscidi et al., 1981) or may be isolated concomitantly with other enteric pathogens, in which case its pathogenic role cannot be assumed (Falsen et al., 1980).

SOURCES OF *CLOSTRIDIUM DIFFICILE*

For most diseases caused by anaerobic bacteria, the epidemiology is straightforward and easily understood. The vast majority of anaerobic infections occur when the host's "normal" endogenous anaerobic flora, common inhabitants of body surfaces, gain access to normally sterile body sites (as in the case of aspiration pneumonia which occurs following the introduction of resident oral anaerobes into the lung). In certain other instances, an exogenous source of anaerobes may be responsible for disease. In most of these instances, the diseases are actually intoxications, caused by exposure to the bacterial toxins, rather than true infections in which the organisms multiply with the host. The clostridial food poisonings are examples. In some specific situations, exogenously acquired anaerobes can cause actual infection, as in tetanus or wound botulism, diseases that occur after the spores of *Clostridium tetani* or *Clostridium botulinum* are introduced into traumatized tissue. In these infections, however, as with most involving anaerobes, introduction of the organisms into normally sterile body sites is an important factor.

The only other anaerobic infection that appears to be somewhat similar in its epidemiological features to *C. difficile*-induced intestinal disease is infant botulism. In this process, it appears that ingestion of exogenous spores of *C. botulinum*, as contaminants of food, may be followed by colonization of the exceptionally susceptible immature intestine, leading to disease mediated by the intralumenal production of the clostridial toxin (Arnon, 1980). It is of note that in all the known instances in which an exogenous, non-living source of anaerobes is of epidemiological importance, the anaerobe involved is a species of *Clostridium*. This is undoubtedly due to the ability of hardy clostridial spores to survive for prolonged periods in many environmental conditions.

Clearly, therefore, there are precedents for both endogenous and exogenous sources of anaerobes as causes of disease. Despite investigations by a number of workers, it is still not known whether endogenous carriage or acquisition from an exogenous source is the usual precursor to *C. difficile*-induced disease.

One problem in ascertaining the prevalence of endogenous carriage is that minor changes in the media used for culture may markedly alter the ability to detect C. difficile. For example, the use of solid media which contain ingredients to enhance spore germination is reported to increase the percentage of positive cultures (Wilson et al., 1982a). Similarly, the addition of an enrichment broth medium may enable the detection of C. difficile from specimens found to be negative when plated on a solid medium (Mulligan et al., 1982). Thus, a major concern about the accuracy of studies to determine the prevalence of carriage of C. difficile is whether the culture media and methods used have been sensitive enough to detect small numbers of organisms. For this reason the relative epidemiological importance of endogenous carriage as a reservoir remains to be defined.

Evidence for endogenous carriage of Clostridium difficile

An intriguing fact is that C. difficile is readily identified as a common member of the intestinal flora of apparently healthy neonates, reported in up to 60% of infants studied (Holst et al., 1981). This microbe is not always, however, a harmless commensal in the pediatric population (Brook, 1980 ; Donta et al., 1981). Interestingly, the first description of the organism, in 1935, was by workers studying the intestinal flora of normal infants (Hall and O'Toole, 1935). Fifty years later, it is still not clear why high counts of these toxigenic clostridia may be harbored with apparent impunity in the intestinal tracts of many neonates, nor is the initial source of neonatal colonization known. Compelling evidence for nosocomial spread among the neonatal population is provided by a study in which fecal specimens of approximately 450 newborn infants were screened daily for C. difficile (Larson et al., 1982). The observed epidemiological patterns of colonization were consistent with person-to-person transmission as well as occasional common source spread. C. difficile was not detected in cultures of vaginal secretions or fecal specimens of 17 mothers of colonized infants; thus, there was no evidence for maternal-child transmission. In a separate study of another nursery population, nosocomial spread was also suggested (Sherertz and Sarubbi, 1982). As noted, the initial source from which the organism gains access to the neonatal population (or any other hospitalized population) is still not known.

In contrast to the high prevalence of intestinal carriage in neonates, fecal carriage of C. difficile appears to be uncommon (detected in less than three percent) in healthy European and North American adults who have not received antimicrobial agents (Larson et al., 1978 , George et al. 1979b; Marrie et al., 1982). This is quite different from the findings of Japanese workers who report higher recovery rates of at least 11.4 percent from fecal specimens of healthy Japanese adults (Nakamura et al., 1981a). Because of previously mentioned variations in methods used to cultivate the organism, it is possible that these reported disparities might be explained by variations in culture techniques; however, there may instead be a real difference in prevalence of gastrointestinal carriage of C. difficile among distinct ethnic populations.

Some evidence against preexisting intestinal carriage of C. difficile as the major mode of acquiring the pathogen is provided by a study of a small group of patients who had fecal cultures performed before, during and after cefoxitin therapy. Although C. difficile was not detected in any pre-therapy specimen, it was isolated from the subsequent fecal specimens (during and/or after therapy) of five of the six patients (Mulligan et al., 1980a). These findings are not conclusive, however, because neither media to enhance spore germination nor an enrichment broth were used, and thus small numbers of the organism in the pre-therapy specimens might have gone undetected.

There has been one study to suggest that another endogenous source of C. difficile might be important. Very high rates of carriage were reported by workers who stated that, using a selective broth medium, they detected C. difficile in nearly three quarters of vaginal cultures from 100 women attending a clinic for sexually transmitted diseases as well as in urethral cultures from all of approximately 40 men with nonspecific urethritis (Hafiz et al., 1975). Urogenital carriage thus might be the reservoir from which colonization of the adult intestine could occur and has also been thought a possible explanation for the high intestinal carriage rates of neonates (who could become colonized during parturition by maternal flora). Unfortunately, other workers have failed to detect C. difficile in genitourinary specimens of males (Piot et al., 1980) or of mothers of colonized infants (Larson et al., 1982); thus the possibility of a urogenital reservoir remains to be confirmed.

Evidence for exogenous sources

Despite the possibility that endogenous carriage may be an epidemiologically important reservoir, there is evidence against this being the only source of C. difficile. A number of studies suggest that disease may occur following exposure of susceptibles to the organism rather than simply as a consequence of proliferation of their previously present floral commensals. Circumstantial evidence is provided by the occurrence of outbreaks or case clustering of pseudomembranous colitis (Kabins and Spira, 1975 , Mogg et al., 1979). In the few instances in which there have been detailed studies of the isolates recovered during outbreaks, there is evidence that a distinctive strain could be identified. In one study, substantial evidence for nosocomial transmission among hospitalized adults is provided by the finding that a strain with distinctive antimicrobial resistance could be recovered from the majority of patients who developed disease while hospitalized on specific surgical wards whereas this resistance pattern was uncommon among isolates from other patients (Burdon, 1982). The majority of isolates recovered during another outbreak also appeared to be of a separate strain, when compared to isolates obtained from other sources (Wüst et al., 1982). Methods used to analyze isolates were agarose gel electrophoresis, crossed immunoelectrophoresis, polyacrylamide gel electrophoresis, and antimicrobial susceptibility. Furthermore, studies in animals indicate that exposure to an exogenous source of C. difficile is important (Larson et al., 1978 , Fekety et al., 1979). The precise methods of transmission which might occur in the apparent nosocomial outbreaks require further study.

Contamination of surfaces in hospital and home environments and carriage of C. difficile on hands and in the intestinal tracts of hospital personnel have been documented (Mulligan et al., 1979 ; Mulligan et al., 1980b; Kim et al., 1981 ; Fekety et al., 1981a ; Sherertz and Sarubbi, 1982). The significance of these potential sources of nosocomial infection remains to be determined. However, the possibility of nosocomial acquisition of C. difficile has led to recommendations that enteric isolation be observed for at least some patients with antimicrobial agent-associated diarrhea and colitis. As discussed below, because diarrhea associated with antimicrobial therapy is a common event and a problem for which C. difficile cannot be implicated as a pathogen in many cases, further study is needed to identify the specific patients for whom isolation would be prudent and to determine the effects of isolation policies on preventing disease.

Other exogenous sources of C. difficile have been described. The organism has been recovered from soil, sand, and mud (Hafiz and Oakley,. 1975). In addition, a variety of animals, including household pets such as dogs, cats, and birds, have been found to harbor C. difficile in the intestinal tract (Borriello et al., 1983b). It seems likely that a person rendered susceptible to acquisition of the pathogen by antimicrobial therapy might be infected after exposure to these animal reservoirs. However, animal to human transmission remains to be documented.

Because other potential enteric pathogens (including some species of Clostridium) are known to contaminate food products (Erickson and Deibel, 1978), contaminated food deserves consideration as a possible vehicle for transmission of C. difficile. If foods were a source of C. difficile, this could provide an explanation for the apparent differences in rates of intestinal carriage among different ethnic groups (whose diets might provide different degrees of exposure to C. difficile-containing foods). There is one report of presumed but not documented foodborne acquisition (Gurian et al., 1982). However, attempts to culture C. difficile from food products have been unsuccessful. In one study, the organism was not detected in approximately 180 food samples, most from the dietetic service of a hospital in which C. difficile-induced disease is common (Oishi et al., 1983).

The need for a typing system

A typing system for C. difficile would be an invaluable tool for further studies of the epidemiology of C. difficile-induced intestinal disease. The relative importance of endogenous versus exogenous sources could be determined. The mode of transmission and the effectiveness of isolation measures in apparent nosocomial outbreaks could be defined. In addition, the common phenomenon of relapse (or reinfection) could be investigated. A variety of typing techniques are under investigation. Preliminary reports of bacteriophage susceptibility and bacteriocin production indicate that these may be useful typing characteristics (Sell et al., 1982). In one previously mentioned study of an outbreak, using a variety of methods, workers were able to identify a distinctive strain (Wüst et al., 1982); these methods should be evaluated further for their utility in a comprehensive system. One of these methods, antimicrobial susceptibility, was sufficient to identify a distinctive strain in the other outbreak (Burdon, 1982) but would not be adequate for typing of all isolates. Serologic typing methods, although not found to be extremely useful in one study (Nakamura et al., 1981b), are still under investigation (Halebian et al., 1983). It is to be expected that with the development of a practical typing system, many presently unanswered questions about the epidemiology of C. difficile-induced disease can be addressed. **For a fuller description see chapter 7.**

ALTERED INTESTINAL MICROECOLOGY AS A RISK FACTOR

In addition to exposure to C. difficile (whatever its reservoir), an alteration in intestinal microecology is an apparently important risk factor for the development of disease. In fact, C. difficile is rarely a pathogen except in the setting of predisposing therapy. There are rare reports of illness in patients with no apparent previous therapy or underlying disorder (Peikin et al., 1980), but in the majority of cases, disease occurs in association with antimicrobial therapy. There has been interest in the possibility that C. difficile might be the causative agent in relapses of inflammatory bowel disease. However, although there is some conflicting evidence, it is not clear that there is a special role for this organism in this group of patients. It may simply be that they, like others, can develop antimicrobial agent-induced illness superimposed on an underlying condition (Trnka and LaMont, 1981 ; Meyers et al., 1981). Other conditions which may predispose to development of disease are reported uncommonly and include cancer chemotherapy, often with agents which may have antimicrobial activity (Fainstein et al., 1981), as well as a variety of apparently rarely associated conditions such as ischemic bowel disease (Wu, 1982), corticosteroid therapy (Greenfield et al., 1981), and Hirschprung's disease (Thomas et al., 1982).

It is not known if there is some common factor in all of these conditions. It seems logical that agents which suppress other anaerobic bacteria and achieve appreciable concentrations in the gut are most likely to alter the microecology so as to allow the acquisition and/or overgrowth of C. difficile. Indeed, the attack rate does appear to be higher in association with drugs which have a potent effect on the fecal flora (Keighley et al., 1979a). However, it is not simply a matter of overgrowth of resistant C. difficile because disease may occur weeks after cessation of therapy, and the pathogen itself is often susceptible to the inciting agent (Dzink and Bartlett, 1980). Studies of antimicrobial treated animals confirm that there is a protective role, often referred to as "colonization resistance" (van der Waiij et al., 1972) of the normal intestinal flora. Furthermore, re-establishment of the normal flora offers some protection to animals with C. difficile-associated disease induced by antimicrobial agents (Fekety et al., 1980). Bacteria which compete with or inhibit C. difficile have been identified in vitro (Fekety et. al., 1980 ; Rolfe et al., 1981), but the in vivo relevance of these bacterial interactions has not been defined (see also chapter 8).

Much remains to be learned about the role of the "normal" endogenous flora. It is only recently that there has been serious consideration given to the consequences of iatrogenic alterations of flora, despite the fact that the theoretical importance has been recognized for a much longer time. For example, it has become clear that antecedant antimicrobial therapy is an important risk factor for the development of many opportunistic infections and that the impact of prophylactic therapy upon the flora is an important concern in the management of the surgical patient as well as the immunocompromised host. Clostridium difficile appears to be a rather unique pathogen in that while rarely harmful in the normal host, the only "compromise" needed to produce a susceptible host is, apparently, an alteration in intestinal microecology. There is as yet no evidence that persons destined to develop C. difficile-induced disease have a distinctive flora or that there is some unique alteration in their flora produced by the inciting agent. At present, it is unclear why some patients who receive an antimicrobial agent become ill while others treated with the same drug remain well. This may simply be a function of exposure to (or carriage of) the organism at a time of susceptibility.

However, there is evidence to suggest that other factors may be involved.

OTHER RISK FACTORS

Because C. difficile may be present in the gastrointestinal tract of persons who have received antimicrobial agents but have no apparent resultant intestinal disease (Mulligan et al., 1980a; Viscidi et al., 1981 ; Marrie et al., 1982), it is clear that there must be some additional factor or factors required for the production of illness. Although there has been little research directed at this specific issue, there are data which may be evaluated for evidence of other possible risk factors.

Studies in which fecal specimens have been cultured quantitatively indicate that disease cannot be predicted based solely on the numbers of C. difficile detected in the specimen (Viscidi et al., 1981 ; Nakamura et al., 1981a). Demonstration of cytotoxin in a fecal specimen is a much better, although not always present indicator of disease (Bartlett et al., 1980a) but, again, presence of disease is not correlated solely with fecal toxin titer (Burdon et al., 1981 ; Lishman et al., 1981a). Obviously if disease does not correlate directly with numbers of organisms (and thus quantities of cytotoxin produced per bacterium), then there must be additional important factors. Indeed, "pathogenic" strains of C. difficile (recovered from patients with documented intestinal disease) often produce larger quantities of cytotoxin than do "non-pathogens" (recovered from asymptomatic persons who have received antimicrobial therapy) (Viscidi et al., 1981 ; Marrie et al., 1982). However, highly cytotoxigenic strains are recovered frequently from the feces of healthy neonates and occasionally from feces of asymptomatic adults (Viscidi et al., 1981 ; Nakamura et al., 1981a). Thus, there must be an additional explanation. These findings also raise the question of why some persons acquire highly toxigenic strains while others are colonized with relatively nontoxigenic organisms.

In addition to the cytotoxin, C. difficile produces a separate enterotoxin (Bartlett et al., 1980a) as well as distinct "motility-altering factors" (Justus et al., 1982). Although there is no evidence to confirm the possibility, it could be that strains vary in their production of these substances and that these may be important independent mediators of disease. In addition, it is possible that other virulence factors will be found. Ability to adhere to the host's gut mucosa is an important virulence factor for many enteric pathogens, a property not yet investigated for C. difficile. Perhaps further studies of the recently recognized substances or of other still unknown virulence factors will provide the explanation for why C. difficile is a pathogen on some occasions but non-pathogenic in other, apparently similar circumstances.

Another consideration is that host defenses or host susceptibility may be important variables in determining whether disease will occur. In one study, cytotoxin neutralizing activity was found in the sera of young adults but less commonly in the sera of elderly subjects (Nakamura et al., 1981a). Although the investigators speculated that this finding might explain the apparently increased risk of disease in the elderly, there are many other possible explanations. In addition, there is no evidence that the serum cytotoxin neutralization confers protection. Antibodies to both cytotoxin and enterotoxin have been detected in sera of patients following C. difficile-induced intestinal disease (Viscidi et al., 1982), but again, the protective effect of this host response is not known. Local immunity, thought to be an important host defense against other enteric pathogens, has not been studied.

PRACTICAL CONCERNS IF CLOSTRIDIUM DIFFICILE IS A NOSOCOMIAL PATHOGEN

Although many questions about the epidemiology of Clostridium difficile-induced disease are not yet answered, available data suggest that it is wise to consider this a contagious disease. Many apparent outbreaks have been reported. One of the most serious of these occurred in two adjacent surgical wards in a Birmingham hospital and led to closing of the wards after nearly 100 patients became ill (Burdon, 1982). Possible methods of transmission were investigated, but at the time sensitive methods for environmental cultures were not available (Keighley et al., 1979b). There are, at present, many reports of clustering of cases and apparent outbreaks involving a variety of patients in many geographic locations, adding to the impression that C. difficile might be a nosocomial pathogen (Kabins and Spira, 1975 ; Mogg et al., 1979 ; Greenfield et al., 1981 ; Bruce et al., 1982 ; Abeyesundere, 1982). Although there is the possibility that these apparent outbreaks might be due to chance or to increased investigation or recognition, it does not appear that this is the case. In two outbreaks, a distinctive strain could be identified (Wüst et al., 1982 ; Burdon, 1982). In a number of institutions, outbreaks or clustering of cases were recognized in a setting of ongoing surveillance (Walters et al., 1982 ; Marrie et al., 1982). In addition, there is the evidence for nosocomial spread of C. difficile among neonates. Thus, although there is not yet proof, there would seem to be sufficient evidence to suggest that nosocmial acquisition of pathogenic C. difficile may occur and that measures to minimize spread of the disease are indicated.

Careful use of antimicrobial agents is one logical measure which might help to minimize the occurrence of C. difficile-induced disease. In the past, little attention has been given to the effects of various agents upon intestinal flora. Especially in institutions where the disease is common, it would seem reasonable to consider the potential for producing this disease when choosing from the available antimicrobial regimens. In addition, as new agents become available, the relative risk of predisposing to diarrhea and colitis should be evaluated.

Prompt recognition and appropriate management of C. difficile-induced disease might also help to minimize nosocomial spread. Because C. difficile may be isolated from feces of many patients given antimicrobial therapy who do not have colitis or diarrhea (Viscidi et al., 1981 ; Burdon, 1982), isolation does not seem necessary for all patients who harbor the organism. Extensive environmental contamination (possibly important in the hospital spread of disease) appears to occur most often in the vicinity of patients who are severely ill, those who are incontinent with extensive, watery diarrhea (Mulligan et al., 1980b). For such patients, enteric isolation seems appropriate and should include physical separation (especially from other patients who are at risk because of antimicrobial therapy) as well as attention on the part of health care providers to avoid transmitting organism on hands or soiled materials. Contaminated articles such as sigmoidoscopes and bedpans should be sterilized or cleaned with sporocidal disinfectants. It is not clear that complete sporocidal disinfection of contaminated hospital rooms is necessary.

Although it is not known if patients who have once had C. difficile-induced disease are at increased risk when subsequently treated with antimicrobial agents, it would seem wise to avoid, if possible, exposing them to agents most likely to predispose to disease and to observe them for signs of the illness should they receive inciting agents.

EXPECTATIONS FOR THE FUTURE

A complete understanding of the epidemiology of C. difficile-induced intestinal disease may bring many benefits. It may be that this common, potentially fatal, and usually iatrogenic illness is, for some patients, preventable or at least predictable. In addition, the answers to the many remaining questions may provide important insights into the interactions of hosts and microorganisms.

CHAPTER 7

TYPING CLOSTRIDIUM DIFFICILE

S. P. BORRIELLO

INDEX

TYPING OF C. DIFFICILE

S.P. Borriello

Introduction

As yet there is no general method for typing *C. difficile*. However, a number of typing methods of use to single centres have been described, and a number of attempts have been made to develop a universal typing scheme.

Biograms

The variation in biochemical properties of isolates of *C. difficile* have been investigated in an attempt to develop a biotyping system. Poxton (1982) found that he could segregate 43 isolates tested into seven different biotypes based on fermentation of glucose, fructose, mannitol and mannose, hydrolysis of aesculin and production of gelatinase. In general when several isolates from the same patient were tested in this scheme they were shown to belong to the same biotype. In a study by Borriello and Stephenson (unpublished observations) of 27 isolates of *C. difficile*, it was shown that reproducibility of test reactions was generally poor (Table 1). All the tests yielding positive results had a reproducibility greater than 80% except for xylose which was only 66.7% reproducible. Similarly all negative tests except aesculin, fructose and glucose gave greater than 78% reproducibility. The remaining tests were only 62-66% reproducible. However, for the purpose of the study undertaken this was considered to be satisfactory provided that each strain was tested in triplicate and that the majority result was taken to be the response to that test.

TABLE 1

Reproducibility of results obtained by subjecting 27 strains of C. difficile to 14 biochemical tests

Test	Positive	Negative	50% variable
Aesculin pH	23 (98.7)*	2 (62.5)*	2
hyd	25 (94.3)	2 (62.5)	0
Fructose	26 (96.5)	1 (66.7)	0
Glucose	23 (92.8)	4 (63.2)	0
Lactose	0	27 (99.1)	0
Maltose	0	27 (99.1)	0
Mannitol	24 (90.7)	2 (78.6)	0
Mannose	23 (94.8)	4 (83.3)	0
Melezitose	18 (85.7)	8 (82.9)	1
Ribose	6 (84.0)	20 (91.8)	1
Starch pH	0	27 (100)	0
hyd	0	27 (100)	0
Sucrose	0	27 (96.6)	0
Xylose	1 (66.7)	26 (99.1)	0

pH = acid production, hyd = hydrolysis, * = % positive or negative of all replicates for all strains.

Working on this basis it was possible to segregate 89 isolates of C. difficile, which included outbreak strains, into two major groups on the basis of fermentation of ribose (Groups 1 and 4) and into 10 groups overall (Table 2).

All of the isolates from infants from hospital K fell into groups 1 and 3, as did an isolate from the environment and one of the mothers (Table 3). In addition all 6 of the isolates from patient EC collected over a period of six weeks and 3 strains isolated from a chair handle and cupboard in the patients room and the ward sluice all belonged to group 1. Patient PT yielded two strains in group 2 that were isolated about three weeks apart, and a strain that was isolated seven months later that is in group 4. It would appear that the patient was colonised by different strains, which is borne out by the fact that the isolates in group 2 were toxigenic and the isolate in group 4 non-toxigenic.

TABLE 2

Biotypes generated by biochemical testing of 89 strains of C. difficile

Test	1	2	3	4	5	6	7	8	9	10
Aesculin hydrolysis	+	-	-	+	+	-	+	+	+	-
Aesculin fermentation	+	+	-	+	+	+	+	+	+	-
Fructose	+	+	+	+	+	+	+	+	-	+
Glucose	+	+	+	+	+	+	+	-	+	-
Mannitol	+	+	+	+	+	+	-	+	+	+
Mannose	+	+	+	+	+	+	-	-	-	-
Melizitose	+	+	+	+	-	-	-	-	+	+
Ribose	-	-	-	+	-	-	-	-	-	-
No. of strains	47	4	2	23	6	1	3	1	1	1

It would seem that biotyping on the basis of biochemical reaction profiles may yield important information on a limited scale, but that the system is insufficiently sensitive for general use. This is highlighted by the fact that nearly 80% of the isolates fell into two groups (Table 2) and that the groups generated failed to segregate cytotoxigenic and non-cytotoxigenic strains which may be different biotypes. Attempts to increase the specificity of the system by increasing the range of test substrates by the use of both the API 20A and API 50 CH test strips have not proved fruitful (Borriello and Cohen - unpublished observations).

A further approach to generating biograms has been the detection of various enzymic capabilities other than carbohydrate fermentation. Borriello and Cohen screened 30 isolates of C. difficile for 120 different enzymic reactions (unpublished data). Of all the tests performed most strains gave similar results and only four tests were found to be of use for differentiation. These were leucine, methionine and L-proline arylamidases and phosphomidase. These enzymic markers could be used to further sub-divide the groups generated by classical biochemical tests.

TABLE 3

GROUPING OF BIOTYPES

Source of strains		Biotype									
		1	2	3	4	5	6	7	8	9	10
Hospital A	Geriatric Ward	4	2	-	1	3	-	-	-	-	-
	Childrens Ward	5	2	-	1	-	-	1	-	-	-
(Rogers et al. 1981)											
	Infant Ward	3	-	-	-	-	-	-	-	-	-
Hospital B		4	-	1	2	-	-	-	-	-	1
Hospital C		5	-	-	2	2	1	1	1	-	-
Hospitals D, E. F		3	-	-	-	-	-	-	-	-	-
Hospital G		-	-	1	-	-	-	-	-	-	-
Hospitals H, I, J		-	-	-	4	-	-	-	-	-	-
Hospital K	Infants	10	-	-	11	-	-	-	-	-	-
(Larson et al 1982)											
	Environment	1	-	-	-	-	-	-	-	-	-
	Mother	1	-	-	-	-	-	-	-	-	-
Hospital L		-	-	-	-	-	-	-	-	1	-
Patient EC	Faeces	6	-	-	-	-	-	-	-	-	-
	Environment	3	-	-	-	-	-	-	-	-	-
Patient PT	Faeces	-	2	-	1	-	-	-	-	-	-

Antibiograms

There have been two published reports on the use of antibiotic sensitivity profiles for typing outbreak strains of C. difficile (Rogers et al. 1981, Wüst et al 1982). In a study of the spread of C. difficile among patients receiving non-absorbable antibiotics for gut decontamination all strains were tested for sensitivity to 20 different antibiotics using a conventional disc sensitivity method (Rogers et al. 1981). Two distinct antibiograms were generated by the isolated strains, differing in sensitivity to penicillin and tetracycline. One of the patients was sequentially colonised by both types. In strains of C. difficile studied by Wüst et al. (1982) it was found that the minimum inhibitory concentrations of most of the antibiotics tested were within a narrow range resulting in most of these antimicrobials being of little use for typing purposes. However, wide variety among C. difficile strains were found in their sensitivities to chloramphenicol, clindamycin, erythromycin, rifampicin and tetracycline. Twelve of the 16 isolates were sensitive to all five of these antibiotics. However, isolates with the same antibiogram were not all the same strain, and included a non-cytotoxigenic strain. It is evident from this study that antibiograms alone would not be sufficiently sensitive for typing outbreak strains of C. difficile.

Soluble protein profiles

Polyacrylamide slab gel electrophoresis has been used to detect soluble proteins of C. difficile and the profiles generated have been used in an attempt to type C. difficile isolates. (Wüst et al. 1982, Borriello and Stephenson, unpublished data). This technique segregated the 16 strains studied by Wüst et al. (1982) into three types, with all of the cytotoxigenic strains exhibiting antibiotic resistance (see above) falling into one group and the 3 antibiotic sensitive strains falling into a different group. The non-cytotoxigenic antibiotic resistant strain was different to the strains in these two groups. Analysis of 44 C. difficile isolates showed that a variety of protein profiles could be obtained. In general outbreak strains gave similar profiles to each other and these profiles differed to those of other outbreak strains (Borriello and Stephenson, unpublished observations). However there were frequent differences between the results of this typing scheme and those of the biotyping scheme based on biochemical reaction profiles (see above). For example some strains that fell into biogroup one (Table 1) were different by protein profiles. This lack of concordance highlighted the poorer sensitivity of typing based on biochemical reaction profiles.

Serotyping

Of the serological typing methods investigated most of the published work is related to crossed immunoelectrophoresis (CIE) techniques (Poxton and Byrne 1981a, Poxton 1982, Wüst et al., 1982). Poxton and Byrne (1981a) and Poxton (1982) have shown that five cell-surface antigens can be extracted from C. difficile (NCTC 11223) with EDTA and visualized by CIE. Two of the antigens have been found in all strains so far investigated. Two of the antigens are also common to C. sordellii and C. bifermentans.

It has been proposed that isolates C. difficile could be serotyped by the detection of 3 of the cell surface antigens, and it has been shown that isolates from the same patient give the same profile (Poxton 1982). Wüst et al. (1982) showed that 15 of their 16 outbreak strains all had the same immunoelectrophoresis pattern. The strain giving a different pattern was a non-cytotoxigenic strain. However, not all the strains that were shown to be the same by CIE were shown to be the same by other techniques (eg. protein profiles as visualized by polyacrylamide gel electrophoresis). This highlights the need for a more complete serotyping system.

Nakamura et al. (1981b) have also investigated serological typing methods, but did not find them to be particularly useful.

Plasmid profiles

Wüst et al. (1982) have shown that of 16 outbreak isolates of C. difficile four different plasmid profiles could be detected by agarose gel electrophoresis of crude lysates. Thirteen of the isolates gave identical profiles, and this major group also included the one non-cytotoxigenic strain. They also investigated 35 C. difficile isolates from geographically different sources and found that 24 strains had no detectable plasmids and that 11 strains all had plasmid patterns that were different to those found in their outbreak strains.

Bacteriocins and Phages

In a recent study Sell et al. (1983) described the isolation of phage from C. difficile that were subsequently used to type a number of their strains. In addition, during the same study inhibitory activity consistent with bacteriocins was noted for 20 strains of C. difficile. The various sensitivities of the 254 isolates of C. difficile tested against preparations of the 10 phage isolated and the bacteriocinogenic like factor are presented in Figure 1. On the basis of host range the authors concluded that none of the phage preparations appeared identical to each other, and that on the basis of the phage-sensitive bacterial isolates, nine distinct phage groups could be detected. Unlike the phage preparations many of the 'bacteriocin' preparations had an identical spectrum of inhibition. However even here 3 distinct ranges of inhibitory activity were apparent. Although the use of bacteriocin typing in conjunction with the phage typing system increased the number of typable strains by 50% it is apparent that many of the isolates could not be typed.

Figure 1

Sensitivity of 254 isolates of C. difficile to bacteriocins and bacteriophage

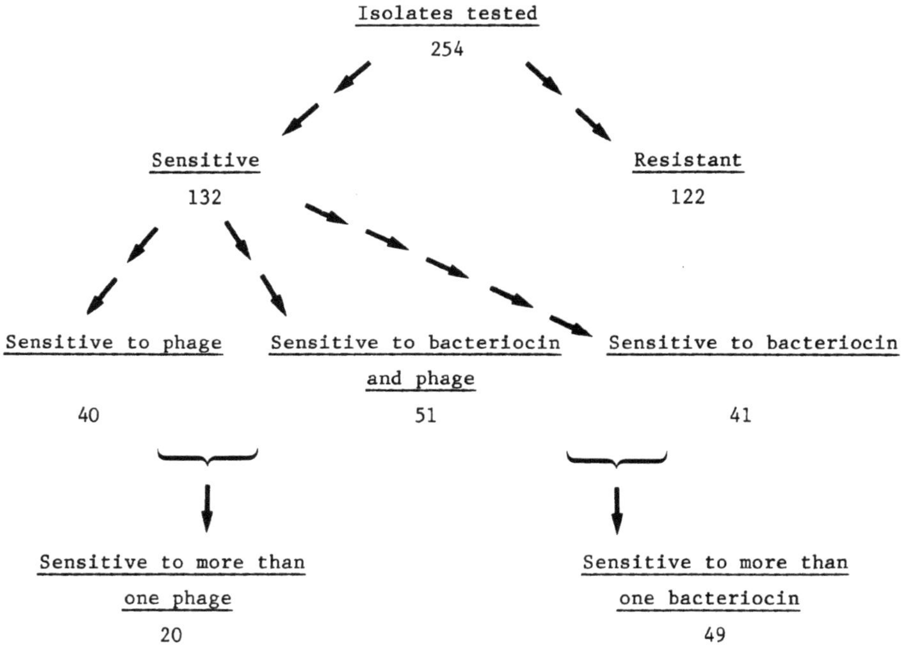

Conclusion

Of all of the typing methods investigated to date it would appear that the phage typing system probably holds out most hope for an acceptable practical typing scheme. The search for a wider variety of phage by different laboratories must be a priority for those interested in this subject. This will increase the number of strains that can be typed and hopefully obviate the need for the inclusion of relative sensitivity to a poorly defined bacteriocinogenic factor(s).

CHAPTER 8

CLOSTRIDIUM DIFFICILE AND COLONIZATION RESISTANCE

Fiona E. Barclay and S.P. Borriello

INDEX

CLOSTRIDIUM DIFFICILE AND COLONIZATION RESISTANCE

Fiona E. Barclay and S.P. Borriello

Introduction

At birth the human intestine is sterile but very quickly becomes colonized with a wide variety of bacterial species, derived formerly from the mother and then from the environment. Eventually, the acquisition of new species ceases and the composition of the flora stabilises so that, in healthy individuals, host and microflora live in harmony. This relationship is important, for although the presence of an indigenous microflora is not essential for life, as is evident from the existence of gnotobiotic animals, it does exert an influence over the normal physiological functioning of the gastrointestinal tract. This includes control of fat absorption and cholic acid hydrolysis, metabolism of bilirubin, protein and urea into ammonia and the synthesis of vitamins from dietary substrate.

The presence of a normal gut flora has also been shown to have an effect on the actual structure of the gastrointestinal tract. In germfree mice and antibiotic-treated hamsters, the surface area of the gut, in particular the caecum, is much larger than in conventional animals. If, however, they are recolonized with their usual flora, the gut eventually reverts to its normal structure.

Perhaps the most important function of the normal, stable microflora is that of a barrier between the host and potential disease-causing organisms. These pathogens may be exogenous or may be members of the normal flora itself, but they are inhibited from causing disease by the complex interactions which make up the stable ecology of an established flora. This inhibition is known as 'Colonization Resistance'. It is only when events occur which alter or disrupt the composition of the flora that this resistance may be challenged. Factors such as health, nutrition and, in particular, administration of antibiotics, are each known to influence the stability of the microflora and this may result in an individual becoming susceptible to infection, either from an 'opportunist' member of the flora or from an exogenous pathogen.

It is generally accepted that in the majority of cases *C. difficile*-mediated disease occurs in this way, usually as a direct result of antibiotic therapy. Most of the antibiotics in general use, with the exception of parentally administered aminoglycosides, have been incriminated in the disease (see chapter 1), including those to which C. difficile is sensitivé, such as vancomycin and metronidazolé, both of which are used in treatment. It is thought that infection probably occurs when the concentration of antibiotic has dropped below that to which C. difficile is sensitive and before the normal flora has had a chance to regain its equilibrium. It has frequently been noted that the majority of C. difficile cultures, including those isolated from subjects with ampicillin-associated diarrhoea, are very susceptible to ampicillin with MIC's of less than 1 μg/ml. Although it was argued that growth of the organism must have taken place once the faecal levels of ampicillin had naturally diminished due to cessation of antibiotic administration, this was not always a satisfactory answer. The dilemma was resolved by the findings of Rolfe and Finegold (1983) who showed that the caecal contents of hamsters with ampicillin-induced ileocaecitis displayed β-lactamase activity whereas those from untreated controls did not. Simultaneous administration of ampicillin and a non-absorbable β-lactamase inhibitor protected hamsters but they developed fatal ileocaecitis once the treatment was stopped. This was due to inactivation of the ampicillin by β-lactamase-producing components of the intestinal flora, thus allowing the normally ampicillin-sensitive C. difficile to establish and cause disease.

In order to understand more about the pathogenesis of C. difficile in antibiotic-associated colitis, a number of studies have been performed using animal models of the disease (Lusk et al., 1978, Fekety et al., 1979, Larson et al., 1980, Dabard et al., 1979, see also chapter 11). It has been established that hamsters treated with antibiotics prior to challenge with a cytotoxigenic strain of C. difficile succumb rapidly to a fatal enterocaecitis. Newborn hares are susceptible to a C. difficile-mediated disease which does not affect adults and it is thought that this may be the consequence of a not yet fully developed intestinal flora. This also applies to human neonates which are regular carriers of C. difficile, albeit asymptomatic in the majority of cases, other mechanisms obviously coming into play to prevent the development of disease.

The above facts indicate that an incomplete normal flora, or one which has been altered in some way, specifically by antimicrobial drugs, will predispose individuals to colonization and/or overgrowth by C. difficile.

Factors involved in Colonization Resistance

When potential pathogens enter the digestive tract they encounter a variety of obstacles which they must overcome in order to cause infection. One of these is colonization resistance and this is conferred in a number of ways, both directly and indirectly. Other factors that can be involved in preventing colonization by a particular organism are anti-bacterial secretions such as bile salts, lysozyme, proteases and gastric acid. The so-called gastric acid barrier is an important factor in controlling any exogenous bacteria coming into contact with the small and large bowel. The gut is also well-serviced with immunological defence mechanisms which include the immunoglobulins G,M and E, secretory IgA and cell-mediated immunity. The role of these mechanisms in controlling the gut flora has not yet been fully elucidated although there is evidence that secretory IgA and cell-mediated immunity do play an active role.

The establishment of an organism in the gut, although dependent upon the negotiation of these environmental hazards, is also affected by the physiology of the organism itself. Factors such as motility, ability to adhere to epithelial surfaces, nutritional requirements and capsule and spore formation may each contribute to the success or failure of the invading pathogen to cause an infection.

The mechanisms controlling colonization resistance are numerous and interacting. Direct resistance may be conferred by ecological interaction, that is, the ecological niches required by the invading pathogen in order to grow and multiply have already been occupied by other bacteria. Disruption of the flora may result in removal of resident bacteria from these niches and replacement by a potential pathogen, either an exogenous or an endogenous 'opportunist'.

Metabolites produced by the many organisms present in the gut may be advantageous in that certain of them can be utilized by other bacteria either directly or indirectly or, conversely, they may be detrimental due to their toxicity. Certain bacteria produce antibacterial substances *in vitro* which are lethal to one or more species and it is assumed that this also occurs *in vivo*. Bacteriocins, for example, are widely produced by both Gram positive and negative organisms and are bactericidal in action. The balance between the number of bacteria and available nutrients is likely to be critical and the most successful species, i.e. those present in the highest numbers, will be those which can most readily utilise the nutrients available.

Indirectly, the intestinal microflora is thought to play an important part in intestinal motility (Abrams *et al*. 1966). Regular peristaltic activity plays a necessary role in clearing the bowel of waste products and, at the same time sweeping away any bacteria not intimately associated with the epithelial surfaces. Impaired motility may lead to a building up of large bacterial populations in the lumen resulting in possible penetration of the mucosa by pathogenic organisms (Formal *et al*., 1963; Kent *et al*., 1966).

Colonization Resistance to C. difficile

A number of studies have been performed to look at colonization resistance to *C. difficile* in animal models and with human material.

We have used both human and animal material in this laboratory to perform a simple *in vitro* test designed to show that the presence of a normal bacterial flora is required for inhibition of *C. difficile* to take place. Caecal contents from both normal, and clindamycin-pretreated hamsters which are known to be susceptible to colonization, were seeded with *C. difficile* and incubated for 72 hours. Results of periodic total counts showed that C. difficile was inhibited to a greater extent by the normal caecal contents.

A similar test was performed using human faeces, an easily attainable source of the bacterial flora to be found in the large bowel. C. difficile was incubated in a 1 in 20 dilution of normal adult stool, heat sterilized stool and a filtrate prepared from normal stool. Total numbers of C. difficile were reduced drastically by normal stool but no such inhibition was noted in the sterilized stool or the filtrate (Borriello et al., 1982). These findings indicate that viable cells must be present in order to provide protection against colonization with C. difficile (Fig. 1).

We have further shown that stools from patients with antibiotic associated diarrhoea fall into the following groups using this test system. Those samples that were not inhibitory to the growth of C. difficile, which presumably represented patients at risk of infection (in fact a patient shown to be at risk by this system subsequently became colonized by C. difficile), and those samples that were inhibitory to growth of C. difficile. The inhibitory samples themselves fell into two groups consisting of those where the sterile faecal filtrate was not inhibitory, implying that they had sufficient inhibitory components of the faecal flora present, and those where the sterile faecal filtrates were inhibitory, showing that a non-microbial component was inhibiting the growth of C. difficile. This inhibition was probably due to antibiotics in the faeces (Borriello et al., 1983[a]).

Infants are frequently colonized with C. difficile in their first week of life (Borriello 1981, Larson et al., 1982, Stark et al., 1982) probably because they still have an incomplete gut flora. It was shown that the faecal emulsion from a breast-fed infant was inhibitory to growth of C. difficile whereas that from a bottle-fed infant was not. The inhibition of the faecal emulsion from the breast-fed infant was retained even when the pH was altered from 5.5 to 8.6, the pH of the non-inhibitory stool (Borriello, 1981). Recent work has shown that the stools of 10 of 12 breast-fed and 4 of 11 bottle-fed infants were inhibitory to the growth of C. difficile.

It is interesting to speculate that one of the reasons for the finding that the elderly have C. difficile infections more frequently (Borriello and Larson 1981) is that they have age associated changes in the gastroinestinal flora that predispose them to colonization with this organism. Preliminary work using the in vitro model has shown that stools from geriatrics with no recent history of antimicrobial treatment are less efficient at inhibiting the growth of the test strain of C. difficile used.

It would be of interest, and of potential therapeutic use, to determine those strains responsible for the protective effect in healthy individuals assuming that the presence of the normal flora in toto is not required. A number of studies have been performed in which the interactions between members of the normal flora and selected pathogens have been investigated. In vitro tests have shown that commensal bacteria, in particular Gram

Fig. 1

Growth of *C. difficile* in faecal emulsions

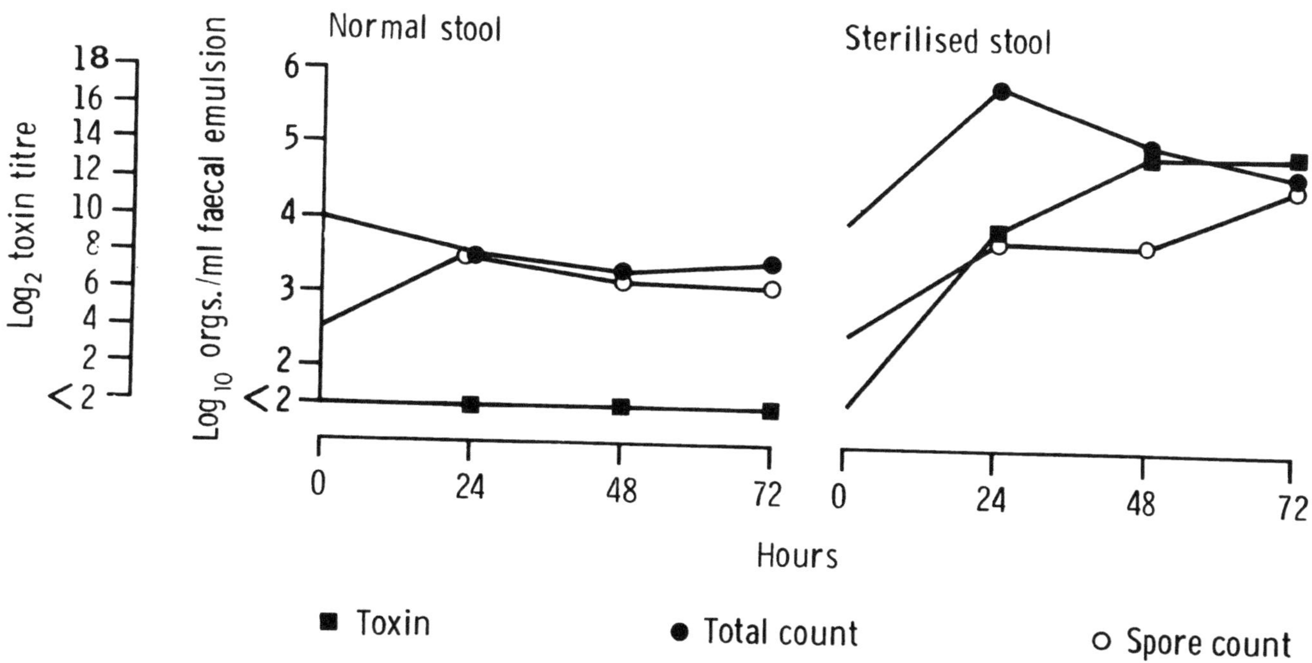

positive organisms, produce antibacterial substances, such as antibiotics and bacteriocins, which effectively inhibit the growth of a range of pathogens (El Sanousi et al., 1978, Sanders, 1969, Mitchell & Kenworthy, 1976, Hentges & Maier, 1970, Hsu and Wiseman, 1967, Sanders and Sanders, 1982). C. difficile is included amongst those investigated. Rolfe and colleagues (1981) tested the in vitro inhibitory capacity of 23 anaerobic and aerobic genera from the normal faecal flora against C. difficile and found that six of the genera showed inhibitory activity, in particular Lactobacilli and Group D enterococci. Malamou-Ladas and Tabaqchali (1982) also demonstrated antagonism between faecal streptococci and C. difficile in vitro and postulated that this may explain the in vivo resistance of the normal intestinal flora to colonization by C. difficile.

Lactobacilli constitute one of the dominant groups of intestinal organisms and are known to perform a number of functions beneficial to the host, such as the synthesis of B vitamins. Natural antibiotics have been isolated from L. acidophilus and L. bulgaricus (Shahani and Ayebo, 1977) which have been shown to be inhibitory to a number of pathogens and also other commensal bacteria. These two species have formed the basis of a commercial preparation (Lactinex) which has been shown to be effective in preventing C. difficile induced ileocaecitis in antibiotic-treated hamsters (Winans et al., 1980) and, significantly, ampicillin-associated diarrhoea in man, (Gotz et al., 1979).

In our own studies, we have isolated from human faeces a species of clostridium, C. beijerinckii which shows an almost totally specific antagonism for C. difficile (Barclay and Borriello 1982). All 50 strains of C. difficile tested were inhibited by this strain and of the wide range of other genera assayed inhibition was evident in only a few cases and generally not as marked as for C. difficile. The nature of the inhibition is bactericidal, and the inhibitor is denatured by heating at 56°C for 30 minutes.

Over the past few years we have become increasingly aware of the presence of strains of C. difficile which do not produce a cytotoxin. When inoculated into clindamycin-treated hamsters these strains do not appear to have the pathogenic potential of the cytotoxigenic strains although they establish and proliferate in the same way. This led to the speculation that the presence of a non-pathogenic strain already well-established in the gut may confer some degree of protection from subsequent challenge with a cytotoxigenic strain. This has proved to be the case (Borriello et al., 1982, Borriello 1983). In order to discover whether protection was due to the exclusion of the pathogenic strain from the mucosa or whether immunological or other mechanisms were at work, the established non-pathogenic strain was removed by treatment with vancomycin prior to challenge with the pathogenic strain. No protection was exhibited nor could it be induced by administration of heat-killed suspensions of the non-pathogenic strain. Attempts to replace the protective strain with other species of clostridia failed and the non-pathogenic C. difficile would not protect against subsequent challenge with a different pathogen,

C. spiroforme (Borriello and Barclay, 1983).

Wilson and Sheagren (1983) have also independently shown that prior colonization of cefoxitin treated hamsters with a non-toxigenic strain increased survival considerably but that simultaneous administration of both non-toxigenic and toxigenic C. difficile did not protect from the effects of the toxigenic strain.

Czuprynski et al., (1983) have used germfree rats as a model for studying the effects of monoassociation with two different strains of toxigenic C. difficile. Of particular interest is the finding that one of the strains, which produced considerably less toxin than the other, colonized the rats with no resulting deaths and no evidence of disease although cytotoxin was detected in filtrates of the caecal contents. We also have a toxigenic strain which does not appear to have the same pathogenic potential as other strains although it yields the same levels of cytotoxin. Clindamycin-treated hamsters remained healthy after inoculation with this strain for the 14 day term of the experiment whereas the 'control' toxigenic strain resulted in death within 48 hours. However, pathology of the caeca from the healthy animals revealed 'possible signs of early disease'. These results imply that other non-pathogenic variants of C. difficile exist and that these should also be studied to see if they exert any sort of resistance to colonization with pathogenic strains.

It is highly probable that to prevent colonization by C. difficile the organisms must be denied access to specific mucosal attachment sites and that this can be achieved either specifically with non-pathogenic variants or non-specifically by re-establishment of normal components of the flora.

A number of workers have looked at the possibility of excluding certain bacteria from the gastrointestinal tract of a variety of animal species. They have attempted to simulate the resistance provided by the full normal flora by inoculating a limited number of species into gnotobiotic mice (Wells et al., 1982) and newly hatched chicks (Impey et al., 1982) and then challenging with Clostridium botulinum and Salmonella typhimurium respectively. The gnotobiotic mice were colonized with two types of flora, one consisting of two or three and the other of eight species. Neither provided protection when challenged with spores of C. botulinum, which proved lethal, but those mice with a complete flora were unaffected. Barnes et al., (1980) established that a mixture of some 23 bacterial strains successfully protected newly hatched chicks from colonization by S. typhimurium although Impey et al., (1982) found that protection using this cocktail was not as reproducible as when a suspension of caecal contents from an adult bird was used. Consequently, they increased the number of bacterial strains to 48, including those strains isolated from chicks who had received the original mixture, and were able to obtain consistent results.

Similar approaches have been made for C. difficile. The entire normal flora, as contained in caecal or faecal material has been shown to confer protection from *C. difficile* in both man and animals. Wilson *et al*., (1980) demonstrated that caecal contents derived from healthy hamsters and administered by orogastric tube and enema to vancomycin-treated animals over a 5 day period was effective in preventing *C. difficile* induced ileocaecitis. Much more significantly, Bowden *et al*., (1981) successfully treated 13 out of 16 patients with pseudomembranous colitis by the administration of faecal enemas. Of the three patients who died, post-mortem examination revealed that two did not have pseudomembranes and one had involvement of the small bowel. Obviously application of faecal material is unpleasant and a preferable approach to the problem would be to prepare a mixture of the minimum components of the total flora required to confer protection. Research is being carried out to this end and it is hoped that such a means of treatment will eventually be available as a more natural alternative to drug therapy.

Faecal markers of colonization resistance

Not all patients who are on antibiotics are susceptible to *C. difficile* infection, and it would be of value to be able to recognize those patients specifically at risk. This could possibly be achieved by use of the bio-assay of growth of *C. difficile* in faecal emulsions (see above). However, this is time consuming and therefore would not be practicable for the majority of laboratories. It would be of value if a readily detectable faecal marker that correlated with the bio-assay could be found. There is a precedent for this sort of approach. Welling & Green (1978) found that a dipeptide, β-aspartylglycine was unique to the caecal contents of germ-free and antibiotic-treated mice. However, when germ-free mice were gradully re-colonized with up to 55 strains of anaerobic bacteria the level of β-aspartylglycine dropped simultaneously (Welling *et al*., 1980). Most interestingly, the strains used had been isolated from the intestinal flora of antibiotic-treated mice showing a high resistance against oral contamination with *Escherichia coli* and, when the germ-free mice were repeatedly challenged with the same strain during re-colonization, it was found that there was an excellent relationship between colonization resistance to *E. coli* and faecal β-aspartylglycine levels. The discovery of such a marker for the simple detection of patients at risk of infection with *C. difficile* would be of obvious value in the prevention of disease, especially if coupled with re-colonization of the gut to re-establish colonization resistance. It is hoped that future work on identifying the components that confer colonization resistance to specific pathogens and on looking for specific markers of colonization resistance will facilitate the detection and management of 'at risk' patients.

CHAPTER 9

CHARACTERISTICS OF THE TOXINS OF CLOSTRIDIUM DIFFICILE

D. M. LYERLY and T. D. WILKINS

INDEX

CHARACTERISTICS OF THE TOXINS OF CLOSTRIDIUM DIFFICILE

DAVID M. LYERLY AND TRACY D. WILKINS
DEPARTMENT OF ANAEROBIC MICROBIOLOGY
VIRGINIA POLYTECHNIC INSTITUTE

INTRODUCTION

The production of toxin by Clostridium difficile was first described by Hall and O'Toole (1935) who noted that subcutaneous injections of cell-free filtrates into guinea pigs caused edema, respiratory arrest, and death. These observations were confirmed two years later by Snyder (1937). Almost 40 years later, Hafiz and Oakley (1976) reported that 5 of 30 strains of C. difficile which they isolated produced very small amounts of toxin that was lethal and necrotizing. They did not study the toxin further, in part because their strains produced only 4 mouse lethal doses per ml. Then, in the late 1970's, the results from a series of studies implicated C. difficile as the causative agent of antibiotic-associated colitis and these findings resulted in the initiation of a number of studies on the toxins of the organism (Bartlett et al. 1977a,1978 a,c,d; Browne et al. 1977a; Larson et al. 1977 , 1978; Larson and Price, 1977; Rifkin et al. 1977, 1978a; Chang et al. 1978a, b; George et al. 1978a,c; Katz et al. 1978; Allo et al. 1979; Willey and Bartlett, 1979; Rehg, 1980).

The cytotoxic nature of the toxins of C. difficile was discovered because diarrhea samples commonly are processed for the presence of cytopathic viruses. The filtrates of feces from patients with pseudomembranous colitis caused the tissue culture cells to become round and detach from the plastic plates. However, unlike viruses, this cytotoxic factor passed through filters that retained viruses and could not be propagated in tissue cultured cells. Thus the activity seemed to be a toxin. Gas gangrene antitoxin was available in these laboratories and investigators soon discovered that this antitoxin neutralized the cytotoxicity. Gas gangrene antitoxin is composed of a mixture of clostridial antitoxins. When the individual components of the gas gangrene antitoxin were tested, only C. sordellii antitoxin was active; however, C. sordellii was not present in most of the human or hamster fecal samples that were cytotoxic. Shortly after these findings, C. difficile was identified as the organism responsible for the cytotoxicity. We now know that these two organisms produce toxins that are very similar if not identical. However, C. sordellii produces much smaller amounts of these toxins, and C. sordellii has not been shown to produce colitis in man or animals.

The early work on these toxins suggested the presence of a single toxin of unusually high molecular weight that was cytopathic, lethal for animals, and which had enterotoxin activity in ligated intestinal loops. Then in 1980, Taylor and Bartlett and later Banno et al. (1981) reported that the enterotoxin activity could be separated from the major cytotoxic factor by ion exchange chromatography. The enterotoxin was also of very high molecular weight, and was present (along with other contaminating proteins) in most of the earlier partially purified preparations of C. difficile toxin.

At the present time, the cytotoxin and enterotoxin are the only known toxins of C. difficile. The enterotoxin is referred to as toxin A because it elutes prior to the cytotoxin, toxin B, during DEAE ion-exchange chromatography.

PRODUCTION AND PURIFICATION OF TOXINS

At the time of the initial purification work, no one knew that the enterotoxin activity and the main cytotoxic activity were caused by two different toxins; consequently, some research groups were working primarily on the cytotoxin (contaminated with some enterotoxin) while others were unknowingly working primarily with the enterotoxin. This made for some confusion that is only now being straightened out. Several research groups reported their preliminary findings in 1978 at meetings, and the general methods for maximal toxin production and partial purification were established by these investigators (Harvie et al. 1978; Taylor et al. 1978; Wilkins et al. 1978; Humphrey et al. 1979; Taylor and Bartlett, 1979; Thelestam and Bronnegard, 1979; Wilkins, 1979).

In 1979, Rolfe and Finegold reported that they had purified the cytotoxin from culture supernatant fluids using ultrafiltration, $(NH_4)_2SO_4$ precipitation, gel filtration on Biogel A 5m, and ion-exchange chromatography on DEAE Sephadex A-25. When analyzed by PAGE and isoelectric focusing, only a single band was detected. These results suggested the absence of contaminating substances in the toxin preparation. However, the results of Sullivan et al. (1982) indicated that cytotoxin purified in this manner contained several contaminating proteins.

Whereas most of the research groups were working primarily with toxin B, our group was unknowingly working primarily with the enterotoxin, toxin A (Aswell et al. 1979; Wilkins et al. 1980). This was a source of some confusion until Taylor et al. (1980) and Banno et al. (1981) reported that there were two separate toxins. Most investigators had been following only the cytotoxicity through the purification procedures. After ion exchange chromatography they were discarding the enterotoxin because that portion of the eluate (which eluted with 0.2 M NaCl) had very little cytotoxicity compared to the material eluting later (with 0.4 M NaCl). Bartlett's group was the first to notice that the highly cytotoxic material which eluted with 0.4 M NaCl would no longer cause the accumulation of fluid in intestinal loops (Taylor et al. 1981). They reported that the enterotoxin (toxin A) was a large molecular weight protein like the cytotoxin and that it formed a dense band at the top of acrylamide gels. They were able to elute small amounts of this toxin from the gels, and noted that antibodies against the eluted toxin reacted with toxin A but did not neutralize the cytotoxicity of toxin B.

Our laboratory recently has purified mg amounts of both toxins to apparent homogeneity as judged by the rigorous criteria of immunoelectrophoresis and polyacrylamide electrophoresis in both gradient and monomeric gels (Sullivan et al. 1982 , 1983). We used a strain of C. difficile that produces very large amounts of both toxins and grew this organism inside dialysis sacks suspended in brain heart infusion (BHI) broth. This procedure is a slight modification of the method used by Sterne and Wentzel (1950) for the production of large amounts of botulinum toxin. The method separates the toxin from the high molecular weight compounds in BHI and results in about a 100-fold concentration of the toxins. The toxins were concentrated further by ultrafiltation and separated from each other by ion exchange chromatography. These steps still left each toxin preparation very impure. The enterotoxin pool was dialyzed against a low ionic strength acetate buffer at pH 5.5. Under these conditions, the toxin was close to its isoelectric point and precipitated while the contaminants remained soluble. For the purification of toxin B, we found that we obtained a better yield if we put the concentrated ultrafiltrate on a hydrophobic interaction column (phenyl-Sepharose) prior to DEAE ion exchange chromatography. The hydrophobic chromatography step also seemed to stabilize the toxin. These chromatography steps removed a large number of the contaminants; however, two contaminants remained which could not be eliminated by isoelectric focusing, hydroxylapatite adsorption, cation-exchange chromatography, or by columns of concanavalin A or glycoboronate. We were finally able to remove them by immunoaffinity chromatography on a gel to which we had coupled antibodies against antigens from non-toxigenic strains of C. difficile. The cytotoxin that passed through this column still had 5 bands by polyacrylamide gel electrophoresis; however, analysis by crossed immunoelectrophoresis showed that the multiple bands were immunologically related. In addition, all of the bands were cytotoxic, indicating that multiple forms of the toxin were present. The existence of multiple forms of the toxin explains some of the conflicting reports about the properties of the cytotoxin. We believe that these multiple forms are the result of limited proteolysis, and we have found them in both culture filtrates and stools from patients (Sullivan et al. 1983).

We have attempted to purify toxins A and B by direct immunoaffinity chromatography, using antibodies that are specific for each toxin. These antibodies readily bind the toxins when they are passed through the gels, but we have not been able to elute the active toxins (Lyerly and Wilkins, unpublished).

PHYSICOCHEMICAL PROPERTIES

A number of physical characteristics of the cytotoxin and enterotoxin have been reported. However, many of these characteristics were determined with culture filtrates and crude toxin preparations. Some of the differences in the reported properties of the toxins thus may be due to contaminants in the preparations.

Both of the toxins are large extracellular molecules. Determinations of the native molecular weights by gel filtration and PAGE have given estimates of 440,000 to 600,000 for the enterotoxin and 107,000 to 550,000 for the cytotoxin (Humphrey et al. 1979; Taylor and Bartlett,

1979; Thelestam and Bronnegard, 1979; Rolfe and Finegold, 1979; Wilkins et al. 1980; Banno et al. 1981; Sullivan et al. 1982). Recently, we have shown that our homogeneous cytotoxin preparation contains 5 immunologically related, cytotoxic proteins which have estimated molecular weights of 70,000, 160,000, 250,000, 280,000, and 340,000, as determined by PAGE in gradient and monomeric gels (Sullivan et al. 1983).

The high molecular weight estimates of the toxins strongly suggests that the toxins are composed of subunits. So far, we have been unable to dissociate either of the purified toxins into subunits, using a variety of combinations of SDS, urea, guanidine-HCl, heat, and reducing agents (Sullivan et al. 1982). The several naturally occurring forms of toxin B may represent different aggregations of subunits, but we have not been able to prove this as yet.

The isoelectric point of the cytotoxin, as determined by isoelectric focusing, has been reported to be 6.2 (Thelestam and Bronnegard, 1979), 5.0 (Rolfe and Finegold, 1979), and 5.4 to 5.6 (Aswell et al. 1979). The latter report, from our research group, was for the enterotoxin, but we did not know that at the time. We have been unable to achieve sharp zones in isoelectric focusing gels for either toxin; they appear to precipitate as they approach their isoelectric points. We believe that the isoelectric point for the cytotoxin is much lower than previously reported, and the fact that this toxin readily precipitates at pH 3.8 supports this view. Unfortunately, most of the activity is lost under these conditions. The enterotoxin precipitates in the pH range of 5 to 5.5, and does retain its activity. We have utilized this property to purify toxin A.

The amino acid compositions of the toxins have not been reported; however, Chang et al. (1981) noted that N-acetyl maleimide treatment reduced the toxicity of the cytotoxin. This suggests that sulfhydryl and dissulfide bonds are necessary for activity. The activity of both toxins is destroyed at 56 C or greater. The cytotoxin, however, is more susceptible to inactivation in acidic and alkaline solutions than the enterotoxin. For example, the cytotoxin is inactivated at pH 4 and pH 9 whereas the enterotoxin is still active when exposed to these conditions (Taylor and Bartlett, 1979; Rolfe and Finegold, 1979; Sullivan et al. 1982).

Proteolytic enzymes, including trypsin, chymotrypsin, and pronase, inactivate both of the toxins (Rolfe and Finegold, 1979; Banno et al. 1981; Sullivan et al. 1982). Rolfe and Finegold (1979) also reported that their cytotoxin preparation was inactivated by high amounts of amylase, and suggested that the cytotoxin might be a glycoprotein. We have not been able to inactivate our cytotoxin preparations with amylase, and the cytotoxin does not bind to gels, including concanavalin A-Sepharose and glycoboronate, which bind most glycoproteins (Sullivan et al. 1982). The cytotoxin is not inactivated by RNase, DNase, or lipase (Taylor and Bartlett, 1979; Rolfe and Finegold, 1979).

The surface charge properties of the two toxins have not been studied in any detail, but some characteristics can be deduced from the general behavior of the two toxins. For example, the cytotoxin binds to anion-exchange resins, including cholestyramine and colestipol, indicating that it is an acidic or neutral molecule (Chang et al. 1978c; Humphrey et al. 1979; Taylor and Bartlett, 1980). The enterotoxin also binds to these resins, but it can be eluted at a much lower ionic strength. The cytotoxin thus appears to be a highly negatively charged molecule at neutral pH, whereas the enterotoxin is not. This is confirmed by the behavior of the two toxins in an electrical field; the cytotoxin moves very rapidly toward the positive electrode, but the enterotoxin barely moves at all. Both of the toxins appear to be relatively hydrophobic proteins since they are retained on hydrophobic gels and can be eluted only with high concentrations of ethylene glycol (Sullivan et al. 1982).

ACTIVITIES AGAINST MAMMALIAN CELLS

A problem with referring to toxin B as "the cytotoxin" is that both toxins are cytotoxic against mammalian cells. Toxin B is referred to as the cytotoxin, however, because it is much more active. Whereas only 170 femtograms of this toxin will cause rounding of Chinese Hamster Ovary cells, nanogram amounts of the enterotoxin are necessary to cause a positive cytotoxic reaction (Sullivan et al. 1982). We considered that the cytotoxicity of the enterotoxin might be caused by contamination with very small amounts of toxin B, but we have analyzed mg quantities of the enterotoxin by crossed immunoelectrophoresis and PAGE without detecting any toxin B. In addition, the cytotoxicity of the enterotoxin is not neutralized by antitoxin made to toxin B.

The cytotoxic titer of the enterotoxin is consistently about 1000-fold lower than the titer of the cytotoxin in culture filtrates. For example, if the cytotoxic titer of toxin B is 10^5, the cytotoxic titer of the enterotoxin is usually about 10^2. Because of the high activity of toxin B in this assay, the cytotoxicity of the enterotoxin is masked unless the two toxins are separated prior to the assay. We have found that small ion-exchange chromatography columns work well for this purpose, and we have used this approach for determining the cytotoxic titers of the two toxins in culture supernatant fluids. In addition, we have recently developed an enzyme immunoassay which is specific for the enterotoxin, and this allows measurement of the enterotoxin without removing the cytotoxin (Lyerly et al. 1983).

We have not been able to isolate a strain of C. difficile which produces only one of the toxins. All of the strains which we have examined either produce both or neither toxin (Lyerly et al. 1983). These findings suggest that the two toxins might be related either at the translation level or by gene regulation; however, the relationship of the two toxins (if one exists) is not known at the present time. The amount of the toxins produced by different strains is quite variable, and isolates produce cytotoxic titers at all levels ranging from 10^{7-8} per ml of culture filtrate to apparently no toxin production at all. The amount of the toxins produced is a relatively stable characteristic of the strain.

The mechanisms by which the cytotoxin acts on mammalian cells have been studied by a number of investigators. Thelestam and Bronnegard (1979, 1980) showed that crude culture filtrates disrupted the actin filament bundles in cells and that this activity was similar to that observed in cells treated with cytochalasin B; however, there was no competition between the filtrate activity and cytochalasin B. They also found that the toxin depressed membrane functions and inhibited the synthesis of protein and nucleic acid, but did not cause immediate cell death. Gurwith et al. (1982) also reported that the culture filtrate inhibited cell division rather than immediately killing the cells, and found that treated cells contained fewer mitotic figures than untreated cells. The intoxication could not be reversed and the cells eventually died within 4 to 5 days without dividing.

The cytotoxin binds to cells even at 0 C, indicating that the binding is not dependent on an active metabolic process or on cell membrane fluidity. However, dinitrophenol inhibits binding so this would argue that energy is required. At normal temperatures the binding appears to become irreversible within a few minutes and trypsinization or the addition of antitoxin does not prevent intoxication (Florin and Thelestam, 1981).

The results of several studies suggest that the cytotoxicity of the toxin may occur via damage to the cell membrane, but since all of these studies used impure preparations of toxins, the results are not definitive. The hydrophobic nature of the cytotoxin is compatible with the idea that cytotoxicity occurs via a toxin-membrane interaction.

Enterotoxins such as Escherichia coli heat-labile enterotoxin and cholera toxin cause fluid accumulation by activating adenylate cyclase. This activation causes an increase in the intracellular levels of cAMP and is associated with a significant fluid response. Several investigators have examined whether the toxins of C. difficile stimulate adenylate cyclase. Vesely et al. (1981) reported that the cytotoxin actually inhibited this enzyme, but that it stimulated colonic guanylate cyclase. Banno et al. (1981) noted that neither of the toxins stimulated adenylate cyclase in rabbit intestinal epithelial cells. More recently, in conjunction with Vesely's group, we have demonstrated that both of the toxins stimulate colonic guanylate cyclase (Vesely et al. 1983). When the two toxins are added together, the stimulation is additive, indicating that the toxins may be binding to different receptors. The stimulation of the guanylate cyclase by these toxins is similar to that observed with the heat-stable, low molecular weight enterotoxins of E. coli and Yersinia enterocolitica. The importance of this stimulation in the disease remains to be determined.

Investigators have attempted to identify a toxin receptor on mammalian cells. Thelestam and Bronnegard (1979) reported that neither addition of gangliosides nor pretreatment of cells with protease inhibited the binding of the cytotoxin to cells. Chang et al.(1980a) tested a number of carbohydrates, sterols, and bile acids to determine whether these substances inhibited the binding of the toxin to erythrocyte lysates. None of the carbohydrates inhibited binding; however, the sterols and bile acids appeared to have some effect. Thus, a lipid component may be involved in the binding, but these results are preliminary and have not been confirmed.

BIOLOGICAL ACTIVITIES IN ANIMALS

The enterotoxin activity in C. difficile culture supernatants was initially described by Rifkin et al (1978b) and Humphrey et al. (1979), who showed that cecal filtrates from hamsters with antibiotic-associated colitis elicited a positive fluid response in ligated rabbit intestinal loops. Following these reports, Taylor et al (1980) and Banno et al. (1981) described the actual production of an enterotoxin by the organism. Higaki et al. (1981) confirmed these observations by showing that culture filtrates of C. difficile produced a positive fluid response in infant mice challenged intragastrically. The fluid response was maximal beginning at 4 h and lasted until 10 h post challenge, after which many of the mice died. This response was different than the responses elicited by other enterotoxins. For example, the heat-stable enterotoxin of E. coli gave a short-term response in infant mice with a maximum at 4 hrs, whereas the response to cholera toxin was considerably slower (Takeda et al. 1978, 1979). In addition, the maximal fluid accumulation ratio (the intestinal tract/body weight ratio) was lower with the C. difficile filtrate than with other enterotoxins.

The availability of more purified toxin preparations has enabled more definitive studies to be performed on the enterotoxin activities of the two toxins. Nanogram amounts of either toxin injected into the skin of rabbits elicit erythematous, hemorrhagic lesions and increase vascular permeability (Banno et al. 1981; Taylor et al. 1981; Lyerly et al. 1982). The enterotoxin also produces a positive fluid response when ug amounts are injected into ligated rabbit intestinal loops, whereas the cytotoxin is consistently negative. The fluid response to the enterotoxin is extremely hemorrhagic and contains mucus, unlike the "rice-water" fluid elicited by enterotoxins such as the cholera toxin (Banno et al. 1981; Taylor et al. 1981; Lyerly et al. 1982). We have found that submicrogram amounts of the enterotoxin produce a positive fluid response in infant mice (Lyerly et al. 1982). The cytotoxin also elicits a positive response in mice; however, the enterotoxin is at least ten times as potent as the cytotoxin in the assay. In addition, at the high doses of cytotoxin which cause a positive response (2.5 ug or greater), more than 50% of the mice are killed. Taylor et al. (1981), on the other hand, have reported that both toxins are negative in the infant mouse assay.

The intracecal injection of C. difficile toxins causes tissue damage which is similar to that observed in hamsters with cecitis. Homogeneous preparations of toxin A, the enterotoxin, produce moderate hemorrhage with fluid accumulation and partially purified preparations of the cytotoxin produce severe hemorrhage without a significant fluid response. The cecal mucosa of hamsters challenged with the enterotoxin show necrosis with acute inflammation, congestion, and hemorrhage. Toxin B, the cytotoxin, produces severe superficial inflammation with congestion and hemorrhage and, in addition, there is some submucosal involvement. Both of the purified toxins are lethal when injected into the cecum of hamsters (Libby et al. 1982).

There are contradictory reports concerning the relative lethal activity of the toxins when they are injected intraperitoneally into adult mice. Banno et al. (1981) reported that 5 micrograms of their preparation of enterotoxin was required to kill mice and that the cytotoxin was not lethal. The enterotoxin preparation of Taylor and Bartlett (1981) was much more potent; only 10 nanograms killed mice. They also reported that although their preparation of cytotoxin was lethal, 400-fold more was required. We found that 150 ng of our enterotoxin preparation and 50 nanograms of our cytotoxin preparation killed mice, so we believe that the two toxins are about equally lethal (Sullivan et al. 1982).

IMMUNOLOGIC PROPERTIES

The discovery of the role of C. difficile in human and animal disease was brought about in part by a fortuitous cross-reaction of C. sordellii antitoxin with the toxins of C. difficile. Initially, it was questioned whether the neutralization by C. sordellii antitoxin was a true serological reaction or whether the neutralization occurred via some "nonspecific" phenomenon. We have found that the U.S. Bureau of Biologics C. sordellii antitoxin reacts immunologically with at least five C. difficile antigens. Two of these are the enterotoxin and the cytotoxin, as shown by cross immunoelectrophoresis using homogeneous preparations of the toxins (Lyerly and Wilkins, unpublished).

In addition to the apparent similarities of C. sordellii and C. difficile toxins, we have found that a few strains of C. perfringens produce a cytotoxin which behaves similarly to the cytotoxin of C. difficile during ion-exchange chromatography, and this cytotoxicity is neutralized by C. difficile and C. sordellii antitoxin (Sullivan and Wilkins 1982) These strains of C. perfringens also produce low amounts of a substance which is positive in the enterotoxin enzyme immunoassay. It is interesting to speculate that the genes which code for the cytotoxin and enterotoxin of C. difficile might be carried by plasmids or bacteriophage that could be transferred among clostridia. There are several reports indicating that strains of C. difficile carry plasmid DNA (Ionesco, 1980; Rossiter et al. 1982; Smith et al. 1981; Wust et al. 1982; Sullivan and Wilkins, unpublished); however, whether the toxin genes are carried on these plasmids has not been determined.

As we stated earlier, the toxins of C. difficile are large extracellular molecules that are consistently present in culture supernatant fluids in a cytotoxic titer ratio of 1000 to 1. In addition, both of the toxins are cytotoxic for every type of mammalian cell tested, although cell lines differ in their sensitivity to the toxins (Donta et al. 1982). These findings suggest that the toxins might be related, and we have attempted to determine any structural similarities between the two toxins with immunological approaches. The most compelling evidence that the two toxins are not related is that antitoxins prepared against each toxin do not neutralize the other toxin (Taylor et al. 1981; Libby and Wilkins, 1982). In addition, we have analyzed homogeneous toxin preparations and monospecific antibody preparations by Ouchterlony double immunodiffusion, tandem crossed immunoelectrophoresis, and fused rocket immunoelectrophoresis. All of these procedures are designed to detect any immunological similarities between antigens. However, we have been unable to detect any spur formation or line deflection by any of these methods. The cytotoxin does not react in the enterotoxin enzyme immunoassay and the enterotoxin is consistently negative in an enzyme immunoassay which we have recently developed for the cytotoxin (Lyerly and Wilkins, unpublished). Therefore, the toxins do not appear to be related immunologically.

ROLE OF THE TOXINS IN C. DIFFICILE DISEASE

The tissue culture assays currently used to diagnose C. difficile colitis detect the cytotoxin of the organism, thus demonstrating that the cytotoxin is produced in vivo. In addition, the finding that neutralizing activity against the cytotoxin can be detected in the sera of PMC patients also confirms the presence of the cytotoxin (Lishman et al. 1981b; Nakamura et al. 1981a). However, because the cytotoxin masks the enterotoxin in the tissue cell assay, the production of the enterotoxin during the disease is not shown by this assay. Aronson et al. (1982a) have recently confirmed the production of the enterotoxin during the disease by showing that a fecal specimen from a PMC patient was positive in ligated rabbit intestinal loops. In addition, they have detected antibodies against the enterotoxin in the serum of the patient. We have confirmed the presence of the enterotoxin in fecal specimens from PMC patients using an enzyme immunoassay (Lyerly et al. 1983). Many investigators believe that the amount of the enterotoxin found in the feces may correlate better with the severity of the disease than the amount of cytotoxin, but this has not yet been tested. The enzyme immunoassay which we developed for the enterotoxin may prove useful for such determinations (Lyerly et al. 1983).

The exact role of these toxins in the disease has not been established, but it appears that both toxins are involved. Vaccination against both toxins is necessary to protect hamsters against lethal C. difficile colitis; vaccination against either toxin alone does not protect them (Libby et al. 1982).

An interesting observation in the study of the pathogenic nature of the organism is that infants may have high numbers of C. difficile and high cytotoxic titers in their stools, yet show no signs or symptoms of disease (Rietra et al. 1978; Gurwith et al. 1981). The cytotoxic titers present in these infants may be equal to or higher than the titers found in adults with severe PMC. When the enterotoxin was discovered we thought that this toxin might not be produced in the infant colon, but we have found recently that infant fecal specimens are positive in the enterotoxin immunoassay. These findings rule out the possibility that the enterotoxin is not produced by the organism in the colon of infants due to environmental and nutritional differences (Libby et al. 1983). Wada et al. (1980) found that neutralizing antibodies against C. difficile cytotoxin were present in colostral specimens from Japanese postpartem women. They suggested that these antibodies may protect infants against C. difficile disease.

SUMMARY

C. difficile produces two known toxins, toxins A and B, which are both cytopathic for all types of tissue cultured cells. Toxin B is referred to as the cytotoxin because it is much more active against mammalian cells than toxin A. Toxin A is commonly called the enterotoxin because it is responsible for fluid accumulation in the gut. Both toxins are lethal, and both appear to be important in the disease process. At least two other species of clostridia produce small amounts of toxins which may be identical to the cytotoxin and enterotoxin of *C. difficile*, but this is not known to be of importance in disease. The mechanisms by which the toxins cause cytopathology or fluid accumulation in the gut is not known, but the mechanism does not appear to involve activation of adenylate cyclase. The cell receptors for the toxins have not been identified; however, the ability of the toxins to act on a variety of cell types suggests that the receptor molecules are ubiquitous.

ACKNOWLEDGEMENT

Our research on the toxins of *C. difficile* has been supported by United States Public Health Service Grant AI15749 from the National Institutes of Health.

CHAPTER 10

INTERACTION OF CLOSTRIDIUM DIFFICILE TOXIN B (CYTOTOXIN) WITH CULTURED CELLS

MONICA THELESTAM and INGER FLORIN

INDEX

INTERACTION OF C. DIFFICILE TOXIN B (CYTOTOXIN) WITH CULTURED CELLS

M. THELESTAM and I. FLORIN

1. Introduction

Two toxins from C.difficile have been described (see Lyerly and Wilkins, this volume), both of which appear important in the etiology of antibiotic-associated colitis (AAC) (Libby et al 1982). Toxin A causes fluid accumulation in rabbit ileal loops and is thus referred to as an enterotoxin, while toxin B is devoid of enterotoxic activity (Taylor et al. 1981; Sullivan et al. 1982). Both toxins are cytopathogenic, i.e. induce morphological changes in cultured mammalian cells. Toxin B, however, is active at very much lower concentrations than toxin A (Donta et al. 1982; Libby and Wilkins, 1982).

Toxin B was discovered as a consequence of the characteristi morphological changes induced in cultured cells by faecal extrac from patients with AAC (Larson and Price, 1977). It was referre to as the cytopathogenic toxin or the cytotoxin of C.difficile. The discovery of toxin A and its separation from toxin B was reported at at a meeting 1980 (Taylor et al. 1980), and the separation method was not published until 1981 (Taylor et al. 1981) and 1982 (Sullivan et al. 1982). Thus all investigations published before 1981 and also some more recent studies were performed with crude toxin preparations, most probably containin both toxin A and B. Therefore some of the effects initially ascribed to toxin B may turn out in the future to be caused by toxin A as recently shown by Rothman and coworkers (1983), or by the combination of toxin A and B. While positive findings with crude preparations are less reliable, negative findings at least allow us to exclude certain activities of the toxin(s). In view of this, and for the sake of completeness the early studies will be covered here in addition to more recent observations made with toxin A-free preparations of toxin B.

To date no report on the mechanism for the cytopathogenic effect of toxin A has appeared. The discussion below will thus be restricted to the process of toxin B-induced intoxication of cultured cells.

2. General characteristics of the cytopathogenic activity of toxin B

More than 20 different lines of mammalian cells have been tested and shown to be susceptible to the toxin (Donta and Shaffer, 1980; Thelestam and Brönnegård, 1980; Chang et al. 1981). These include fibroblasts, epithelial-like cells and neuroblastoma cells. The morphological effect induced in monolayer cultures of fibroblasts has been termed "actinomorphic". The cytoplasm contracts around the cell nucleus, leaving long processes radiating from the rounded cell body (Chang et al. 1978a; Thelestam and Brönnegård, 1980). At later stages (after 24-48 h) these processes detach and the cells **all appear round** (Florin and Thelestam, 1981). In contrast monolayer cultures of epithelial-like and neuron-like cells after treatment with toxin only round up with no projections (Donta and Shaffer, 1980; Thelestam and Brönnegård, 1980; Gurwith et al. 1982). Both these morphological effects are referred to as the cytopathogenic effect (CPE) of the toxin B. Expression of the CPE as either an actinomorphic change or a cell rounding probably reflects differences in cytoskeletal organization in different cell types rather than differences in the mode of action of the toxin.

Upon addition of toxin to monolayer cultures the CPE appears after a latency period. Its length is dependent on the temperature and on the amount of toxin added (Florin and Thelestam, 1981), but it is not shorter than approximately 45 minutes (Chang et al. 1979b; Florin and Thelestam, 1983). The final level of CPE appearing in toxin-treated cells (i.e. per cent cells with CPE) is dependent on the dose of toxin and the exposure time in relation to the number of cells (Florin and

Thelestam, 1981).

Cells in suspension culture (which are already rounded) do not change morphologically after toxin-treatment, as viewed under the light microscope. However, Gurwith and coworkers (1982) reported growth inhibition of human cervix carcinoma (HeLa) and mouse adrenocortical tumour (Y1) cells in suspension. Likewise the growth in suspension of ascites sarcoma cells as well as of human lymphoblastoid cells is inhibited (Florin and Thelestam, unpublished).

Although mammalian cells in general are sensitive to the toxin, other eukaryotic cells such as some yeasts were found completely insensitive (Florin and Thelestam, unpublished). The growth of several species of gram-positive and gram-negative bacteria was also not affected (Florin and Thelestam, unpublished).

3. Toxin receptors on the cell surface?

Cultured cells are irreversibly intoxicated after short (30 s) toxin treatments followed by thourough rinsing to remove unbound toxin (Donta and Shaffer, 1980; Thelestam and Brönnegård, 1980; Florin and Thelestam, 1981). Thus the toxin is likely to bind to (specific?) receptors on the cell surface. Toxin binding to fibroblasts is independent of temperature and seems firm. After incubation of toxin-treated cells in medium for 24 h at 4°C the toxin still remained located at the cell surface, since the usual CPE developed upon cell warming (Florin and Thelestam, 1981).

Which is the cell surface structure responsible for binding of the toxin? The putative receptor has not yet been identified although it should be a ubiquitous component present on all cell membranes. Only a few preliminary reports have focused on this problem. Most of them present negative findings and some contradict each other. The approaches to receptor identification include studies of (i) receptor blockade by various lectins, (ii) blocking of the CPE after pretreatment of the toxin with various cell membrane components, and (iii) removal of receptors by pretreatment of cells with various enzymes.

Using lectins Levy and Onderdonk (1981) found that wheat germ agglutinin (WGA) reduced the CPE in toxin-treated monkey kidney fibroblasts, whereas phytohemagglutinin (PHA) was without effect. Donta and Shaffer (1980) found concanavalin A (con A) not to be protective in epithelial-like cells. On the other hand we found that preincubation of human fibroblasts with con A and ricin caused a delay of the CPE (Florin and Thelestam, 1983). Five other lectins, including WGA and PHA, were not protective. Results with lectins, however, should be interpreted with caution in terms of specific receptor blockade. We consider such a blockade less conceivable in our system since (i) a CPE did eventually develop in cells pretreated with the protective lectins before the short binding step, and (ii) the lectins delayed the CPE even upon addition after binding of the toxin (Florin and Thelestam, 1983). At least con A is known to interfere with endocytosis in various cells (Middlebrook et al. 1979; Wortmann et al. 1979; Delfini et al. 1982). Thus our findings, and perhaps also those of others who have used lectins, might be better explained as an interference with the cellular internalization of the toxin (see section 5).

Chang and coworkers (1980a) determined binding of the toxin to erythrocyte ghosts indirectly, by measuring loss of cytopathogenic activity from toxin solutions after contact with the erythrocytes. Inhibition of binding was reported with certain sterols and bile acids, whereas a number of monosaccharides, amino sugars and neuraminidase were ineffective. Thus a lipid component was suggested to play a role in toxin binding to erythrocytes. Donta and Shaffer (1980) could not inhibit intoxication of epithelial-like cells with gangliosides. Thelestam and Brönnegård (1980) reported that preincubation of the toxin with high concentrations of cholesterol, gangliosides or lecithin did not abolish its subsequent activity on fibroblasts. Neither was the characteristic cytopathogenic response altered by preincubation of the cells with a phospholipase C hydrolysing all major membrane phospholipids. Thus at least on the surface of cultured cells a lipid receptor seems less likely. The assay system used by Chang and coworkers is not entirely satisfactory for binding studies since both membrane faces are accessible in ghost preparations, and since various membrane components might be abnormally exposed after lysis.

Recently Griffin and collaborators (1982) were able to retard the toxin effect in baby hamster kidney fibroblasts with fetal calf serum, fetuin and thyroglobulin. Using fetal calf serum this finding was confirmed with lung fibroblasts in our laboratory. Dialysed papain digests of fetuin, containing 98% of the original sialic acids but only 1% of the protein, also retarded cytotoxicity (Griffin et al. 1982). These results imply that the recognition site on cells might contain sialic acid. However, we recently observed that the CPE is inhibited by the presence of various nucleotides during the binding step (Florin and Thelestam, unpublished). Whether this means that cationic components are exposed at the receptor site or that the toxin itself binds the nucleotides remains to be seen. Nucleotides inhibit the action of diphtheria toxin by binding to a so called P-site on the toxin (Lory and Collier, 1980).

All attempts so far at clarifying the nature of the receptor can be criticized for using only indirect binding assays. An unambiguous identification of the receptor must await preparation of the highly purified labeled toxin needed for direct binding assays.

4. Effect of the toxin on the cell membrane?

The cell membrane has been proposed as **the main target for th** toxin. Rothman and Brown (1981) reported a decrease in the intracellular level of K^+ in HeLa cells within 1 h of toxin exposure, and an inhibition of the uptake of amino acid after 1 h. Recently these experiments were repeated with purified toxin. HeLa cell rounding was found to occur before any effects on membranes could be measured (Rothman et al. 1983 and personal communication).

In a preliminary report (Madsen and Knoop, 1981) the toxin was claimed to cause a release from prelabelled Y1 cells of ^{14}C-α-aminoisobutyrate after 5 min and of ^{3}H-uridine nucleotides after 1 h toxin exposure. We were not able to confirm these results with either Y1 cells or lung fibroblasts, as tested according to the same methods (Thelestam and Möllby, 1975, 1976) as used by Madsen and Knoop. Neither a partially purified toxin preparation nor even a crude one caused any significant release of amino acid after 30 min, or nucleotides after 24 h exposure (Thelestam and Brönnegård, 1980 and unpublished). The intracellular level of ATP remains constant during the latency period (Florin and Thelestam, 1982), a finding also not supporting membrane damage. More recently Gurwith et al (1982) reported that ^{51}Cr-labelled HeLa cells released less than 5% of the label after 24 h toxin exposure, and also concluded that the cell membrane remains intact.

The morphological changes in C.difficile toxin treated cells (which remain rounded and intact for at least 3 days) are entirely different from the cellular changes typically caused by membrane damaging toxins (Thelestam and Möllby, 1976; 1983). One of the characteristics of such changes in monolayer cells is the intactness of the microfilament bundles (Osborn and Weber, 1977). Moreover C.difficile toxin-treated cells exclude the vital dye trypan blue even after 24 h of toxin exposure (Donta and Shaffer, 1980; Thelestam and Brönnegård, 1980; Gurwith et al. 1982). This is another indication of the lack of membrane permeabilization, since uptake of trypan blue is a measure of membrane damage rather than of cell death (Thelestam and Möllby, 1983).

Lee and Thomsen (1982) demonstrated crenation of guinea pig erythrocytes after 2 h of toxin exposure, and suggest membrane injury to be the cause. However, the toxin was evidently not hemolytic to these cells. Neither is it lytic to human, sheep or rabbit erythrocytes (Thelestam and Brönnegård, 1980). Usually membrane damaging toxins are hemolytic. The crenation is more likely to depend on an effect on the cytoskeletal elements conferring on red cells their typical disc shape. Similarly the ultrastructural changes in type and distribution of amnion cell surface microvilli (Chang et al. 1979b) as well as the reduction in number of microvilli on chinese hamster ovary cell surfaces (King and Murray, 1981) might be related to submembraneous cytoskeletal alterations (see section 6). Alternatively the observed rearrangements of microvilli could accompany a lateral redistribution in the membrane plane of the putative toxin-receptor complex. The multivesicular bodies detected in the plasma membranes after toxin exposure (King and Murray, 1981) could possibly represent endocytotic vesicles related to toxin internalization.

In conclusion, a membrane damage (permeabilization) by the C.difficile toxin B does not appear likely. This conception is consistent with the finding that the toxin must be internalized to exert its cytopathogenic action (see section 5).

5. Cellular internalization of the toxin

During the past few years a growing number of intracellularly acting protein toxins have been shown to be internalized in target cells by (receptor-mediated) endocytosis (Middlebrook and Kohn, 1981). Regarding the C.difficile toxin B this question seems sofar to have been addressed only by our group. A summary of our findings (Florin and Thelestam, 1983) using a highly purified preparation of the toxin follows below:

(i) The toxin disappears rapidly from the fibroblast surface after binding. This was shown by neutralization with antitoxin and by inactivation with trypsin of the toxin bound to the cell surface. Antitoxin or trypsin had to be added within one tenth of the latency period to afford significant protection against intoxication. After this time the toxin has apparently entered the cell.

(ii) The CPE is prevented by inhibitors of the energy metabolism, and by keeping the toxin-treated cells at $0^{o}C$ or transferring them to $0^{o}C$ before the end of the latency (Florin and Thelestam, 1981). Since endocytosis depends on metabolic energy and fluid membranes these results are also consistent with a cellular internalization of the toxin.

(iii) The CPE is prevented by lysosomotropic agents. Upon addition after toxin binding but within one fifth of the latency period ammonium chloride (10 mM) or chloroquine (0.1 mM) protected most of the cells against CPE. Lysosomotropic agents are believed to trap internalized (endocytosed) material in endocytotic vesicles or lysosomes by raising the pH (Maxfield, 1982). Inhibition of biological effect by lysosomotropic agents is therefore generally considered to indicate internalization by endocytosis of the active agent (Middlebrook and Kohn, 1981).

(iv) At pH 4.5, but not at physiological pH, the toxin induced K^+-release from preloaded lipid vesicles. In analogy with recent findings for the diphtheria and tetanus toxins (Boquet and Duflot, 1982) the formation by the toxin of channels in these artificial membranes may be inferred. The result is suggestive of a toxin transfer from acid endocytotic vesicles or lysosomes to the cytosol through similarly formed channels.

In conclusion, all evidence now available to us supports a cellular internalization of the toxin by endocytosis.

6. Intracellular target for toxin action?

What takes place in the toxin-treated cell before appearance of the CPE? Assuming our concept of toxin internalization is correct, the step after toxin transfer from endocytotic vesicles or lysosomes should involve interaction with an intracellular primary target, leading to expression of the intoxication as the characteristic CPE. This target has not yet been identified, but the results up to now allow us to exclude certain targets and to propose a likely target.

The toxin does not have any primary effect on the synthesis of DNA, RNA or protein. Macromolecular synthesis is indeed gradually decreased in HeLa cells (Rothman and Brown, 1981; Rothman et al. (1983) and in lung fibroblasts (Florin and Thelestam, 1981), but this takes place clearly after appearance of the CPE in 100% of the cells. The uptake of macromolecule precursors was reported by the same groups to be gradually depressed in toxin-treated cells, but also these effects are secondary to the CPE. Since the intracellular level of ATP was unchanged well after 100% CPE was reached (Florin and Thelestam, 1982) toxin-interaction with the ATP-generating machinery seems unlikely.

Vesely and coworkers (1981) studied toxin effects on enzyme activities in microsomal preparations from hamster colonic tissue. They report a lack of effect on the Na^+-K^+-ATPase activity, but stimulation of guanylate cyclase and inhibition of adenylate cyclase upon incubation of such subcellular fractions with toxin for 10 min. Cultured hamster fibroblasts incubated with the toxin for 24 h showed a threefold increase in cGMP levels (Vesely et al. 1981). Donta and Shaffer (1980) report a lack of activation of adenylate cyclase or increase in steroid production by Y1 cells. These authors do not comment on any possible inhibition of these activities.

The findings of Vesely and collaborators suggest that the toxin might somehow affect the cyclic nucleotide regulating system. Unfortunately the authors do not report on the levels of cellular cGMP after shorter toxin-treatments. Thus it is not clear whether the putative guanylate cyclase activation in intact cells and subsequent elevation of cGMP is primary or secondary to the CPE. Moreover some doubt has recently been expressed as to the purity of the toxin used in these experiments (Sullivan et al. 1982). Guanylate cyclase will indeed become a good candidate for **a primary toxin target if the** cGMP levels in intact cells can be shown to increase clearly before appearance of the CPE upon treatment with highly purified toxin B.

The CPE of the toxin is rather different from the morphological effects caused by other bacterial cytotoxins acting intracellularly, or by the cytolysins acting on the cell membrane. The conspicuous actinomorphic effect, as viewed both by light and scanning electron microscopy, is closely similar to that induced by the microfilament-interacting cytochalasins (Miranda et al. 1974). This observation led us to a working hypothesis that microfilaments might be attacked by the toxin. Indeed a disorganization of the straight microfilament bundles could be demonstrated in toxin-treated fibroblasts by immunofluorescence with anti-actin antiserum (Thelestam and Brönnegård, 1980). Most of the actin was condensed around the cell nuclei in a non-filamentous form and similar changes occurred in cells treated with cytochalasin B. Parallelling the toxin-induced effect on microfilaments another cytoskeletal component of fibroblasts, the cell surface protein fibronectin, was lost (Ahlgren et al. 1983). The loss of fibronectin is likely to be a secondary phenomenon in the intoxication process since the CPE was induced also in mutant fibroblasts completely lacking fibronectin (Ahlgren et al. 1983). However, the fact that also cytochalasin B causes loss of fibronectin concomitantly with microfilament disorganization (Kurkinen et al. 1978) lends further support to the analogy with the C.difficile toxin. Also Donta and Shaffer (1980) pointed out similarities in the effects induced by the toxin and by cytochalasins.

Our observations concerning the cytoskeletal disorganization by the toxin were originally made using partially purified toxin. More recently they were confirmed with a highly purified toxin (Florin, Thelestam and René Norberg, unpublished). Moreover Wedel and collaborators (1983) very recently showed that purified toxin B induces disorganization of the actin-containing myofilament bundles in rabbit smooth muscle cells. As monitored by transmission electron microscopy this effect occurred concomitantly with appearance of the CPE, while all other cell organelles still appeared unaffected. These observations give further support to the idea that microfilaments are attacked at an early stage of the intoxication process.

In the light of these data we propose microfilaments as a likely primary intracellular target for the action of toxin B. The toxin could interact with any of the large number of factors which appear to be involved in the complicated regulation of microfilament structure and function (Weber and Glenney, 1982). Possibly the toxin can be used as a new tool in this fascinating area of cell biology.

7. Which cellular processes are required for expression of the CPE?

A different approach to identification of the intracellular toxin target is to clarify whether expression of the CPE requires any specific cellular process. We found that in fibroblasts intoxication proceeds as usual in the absence of DNA-, RNA- and protein-synthesis (Florin and Thelestam, 1983), as also reported by Donta and Shaffer (1980) concerning protein synthesis. By contrast the CPE was not expressed in the absence of metabolic energy (Florin and Thelestam, 1981 and 1983).

Of course energy is required for the formation of endocytotic vesicles. However, the CPE was prevented also by addition of inhibitors of the energy metabolism after the endocytotic step. The need for energy at this stage is conceivable if transfer of the toxin to the cytosol is assumed to occur by a pH-dependent channel formation (see section 5). Maintenance of a much lower pH in endocytotic vesicles and lysosomes than in the cytosol, i.e. pH-gradients, requires metabolic energy (Schneider, 1981).

The CPE in fibroblasts was completely blocked by addition of 2,4-dinitrophenol even immediately before the CPE was to develop (Florin and Thelestam, 1981). Thus it appears possible that energy is needed also for some reaction taking place after transfer of the toxin to the cytosol. If the CPE involves a hypercontraction of the microfilaments energy would be required at this late stage. Another conceivable energy-requiring step could involve enzymatic reaction(s) among the components regulating the microfilament structure/function.

8. Fate of intoxicated cells after expression of the CPE

Although the *C.difficile* toxin B is generally referred to as a cytotoxin its effects in cell cultures, as pointed out by Donta and Shaffer (1980), are not associated with classical cytotoxic, i.e. degenerative, changes. In epithelial-like cells the CPE rather looks cytotonic, i.e. cell rounding associated with adenylate cyclase activation. However, this toxin as already mentioned does not stimulate adenylate cyclase. Moreover it causes morphological changes in all cells studied, in contrast to the cytotonic enterotoxins of *V.cholerae* and *E.coli*. The effect of the *C.difficile* toxin then can not be described as cytotonic according to the definition given by Keusch and Donta (1975).

If the toxin is neither cytotonic nor a classical cytotoxin, what is it? Are the intoxicated cells dead or alive? What happens to them upon continued incubation in growth medium at 37°C?

After 24 h with manifest CPE intoxicated fibroblasts still showed a residual metabolism in the form of RNA- and protein synthesis (Florin and Thelestam, 1981). This was also noted in HeLa cells (Rothman and Brown, 1981). However, the DNA-synthesis in fibroblasts was completely inhibited in 24 h (Florin and Thelestam, 1981). After about the same time the toxin caused a clear decrease in mitotic figures in both HeLa and Y1 cells (Gurwith et al. 1982). Cells trypsinized and reseeded after a 24 h toxin exposure did not proliferate (Thelestam and Brönnegård, 1980; Gurwith et al. 1982). Toxin-treated cells were also unable to clone in soft agar (Gurwith et al. 1982), a natural consequence of inhibition of the cell division.

As mentioned above intoxicated cells exclude trypan blue, indicating intact cell membranes and that they are "viable" according to the classical physical definition of cellular life and death. Intoxicated cells give the impression of being in a resting state since they remain firmly attached to the culture well despite the changed morphology. However, according to a genetic definition, i.e. based on ability to proliferate, such cells must be considered dead. Indeed, intoxicated cells begin to deteriorate in 3-4 days as seen in the light microscope (Florin and Thelestam, 1981).

All these observations are consistent with our hypothesis of microfilaments as target for the toxin. Microfilaments are needed for a number of cellular processes, among which are cell spreading on solid surfaces, cell motility, contractility and cytokinesis (Wessells et al. 1971). Microfilaments also confer on cells their typical shape. Anchorage-dependent cells need to be able to spread out in order to synthesize DNA and to divide (Ben-Ze´ev et al. 1980). Cells cultured in suspension need contractility and cytokinesis for their division (Wessells et al. 1971).

For comparison it may be interesting to note that cytochalasin B-treated cells can be held for several days in a resting state, strongly resembling that of C.difficile toxin B-treated cells: they remain rounded but attached, and do not divide. Upon removal of the cytochalasin all microfilament-dependent functions are restored (Wessells et al. 1971; Thelestam and Florin, unpublished). By contrast the C.difficile toxin B-treated cells have irreversibly lost these functions.

9. Conclusion

Based on the currently available pieces of information concerning the mechanism of action of the C.difficile toxin B our present view of the cellular intoxication process can be summarized as follows:

The toxin binds rapidly to unidentified receptors on the cell surface and is internalized in endocytotic vesicles which may fuse with lysosomes. At the low intravesicular pH the toxin forms membrane channels permitting transfer from the vesicles to the cytosol. The subsequent intracellular events are independent of synthesis of DNA, RNA and protein, but depend on metabolic energy. These events involve an attack on microfilaments, either directly by binding to actin, or more probably via regulating components. The shape of monolayer cells is changed due to hypercontraction of the microfilaments or their collapse by depolymerization or by some other disorganization of their supramolecular state. This leads to loss of fibronectin, rearrangement of surface microvilli and loss of all intracellular and membrane-associated microfilament-dependent functions. Transport processes and macromolecular synthesis are gradually depressed, conceivably since they depend on a functioning network of cytoplasmic microfilaments. Mitosis is inhibited in the absence of DNA-synthesis Finally the cells deteriorate because of a lack of the proteins needed for the overall maintenance of intact cells.

10. Future aspects

There are many questions to answer in order to understand the intoxication process in all its molecular details. First of all: what is the chemical structure of the toxin? Is it composed of an intracellularly active A-fragment and a B-fragment(s) responsible for the receptor-binding, in analogy with several other intracellularly acting toxins? Will also this toxin turn out to contain a hydrophobic domain which is exposed at low pH, allowing toxin insertion into membranes? What is the nature of the receptor? Is the toxin-receptor complex clustered in the membrane plane before internalization? Are coated pits involved in the endocytosis? What is the significance of our observation that the CPE is inhibited by nucleotides, a phenomenon also described for diphtheria toxin (Middlebrook and Dorland, 1979)?

Which is the irreversible intracellular step? Is the toxin enzymatically active as are other intracellularly acting toxins? If so, which is the substrate for its action? One obvious way of addressing this question is the investigation of a possible post-translational modification of proteins in intoxicated cells, with special consideration given to components involved in microfilament regulation. Preliminary observations in our laboratory indicate a stimulation of the CPE at elevated intracellular levels of Ca^{++} as induced with the Ca ionophore A 23187. By contrast Zn^{++} blocks the CPE at any stage during its development (Florin and Thelestam, unpublished). These two ions have been implied as antagonists in the function of calmodulin (Brewer, 1980), a protein participating in microfilament regulation. Thus it will be interesting to examine whether the toxin modifies calmodulin, and if other calmodulin antagonists interfere with expression of the CPE.

It is also exciting to speculate about the possible relationship between the C.difficile toxin B and the toxins produced by other clostridia, particularly the neurotoxins from C.tetani and C.botulinum. The extremely low LD_{50}ies of these toxins suggest an enzymatic activity, which is reasonable also for the C.difficile toxin. Tetanus toxin was recently shown to contain a hydrophobic domain, permitting its insertion in membranes at low pH (Boquet and Duflot, 1982). Very little is known about the action of these toxins at the molecular level. However, it is clear that they prevent the release of transmitter substances at nerve synapses. This is attained by inhibition of the exocytosis of vesicles containing the transmitters. Exocytosis, like endocytosis, should depend on functioning microfilaments. Indeed tetanus toxin has been shown to interact with actomyosin-like proteins, i.e. the same components that build up microfilaments (Stephen and Pietrowski, 1981).

Very speculatively: all three clostridial toxins might affect the same contractile proteins. Their differential effects *in vivo* could then depend on different specificities of the receptors involved in the transport of these toxins to their respective targets. Variations at the cellular level could be due to minor variations in intracellular substrate specificities as well as to specific properties of the cells attacked. In view of this idea it might be worthwhile to find out whether the *C.difficile* toxin could affect transmitter release in any of the *in vitro* synaptosomal systems which are now being developed.

In conclusion, the rapidly expanding research on *C.difficile* and its toxins seems to open up new interesting perspectives both in toxinology and in basic cell biology.

ACKNOWLEDGEMENTS

We appreciate stimulating discussions with Patrice Boquet and John Middlebrook. Thanks to Sara Rothman for providing unpublished data. We are grateful to Birgit Sehlberg for skilful and rapid typing of the manuscript. Investigations carried out in our laboratory were supported by the Swedish Medical Research Council.

CHAPTER 11

ANIMAL MODELS OF CLOSTRIDIUM DIFICILE INFECTION

R. FEKETY

INDEX

ANIMAL MODELS OF CLOSTRIDIUM DIFFICILE INFECTION

ROBERT FEKETY

INTRODUCTION

Pseudomembranous colitis caused by *Clostridium difficile* can be a serious complication of therapy with many of our most useful antibiotics (Bartlett 1979 , Fekety *et al*. 1979). While attention was called to this side effect about ten years ago by cases that occurred after use of lincomycin or clindamycin, it is now apparent the syndrome can be precipitated by treatment with almost all antibiotics used for treatment of serious infections. Important clues to the pathogenesis of the disease were determined by study of animal models of the disease. Antibiotic-induced enterocolitis in hamsters was a particularly useful model (Silva, 1979), and studies with it established that the disease is caused by antibiotic-induced overgrowth of toxigenic *Clostridium difficile* (Bartlett *et al*. 1979b, Larson *et al*. 1978).

The key observation was made by Small, who reported that Golden Syrian hamsters given a single subcutaneous injection of lincomycin often died with enterocolitis (Small, 1968). Subsequently, several other groups showed that clindamycin-treated hamsters also developed the syndrome, and that other antibiotics, including the cephalosporins, could cause a similar disease (Lusk *et al*. 1978, Bartlett *et al*. 1978c, Fekety *et al*. 1979, Ebright *et al*. 1981). Eventually it was found that a cytotoxin detectable by its effects on cell-cultures was present in the stools of hamsters with the disease (Rifkin *et al*. 1977, Larson and Price 1977, Bartlett *et al*. 1978a), and that the toxin could be neutralized by either polyvalent Clostridial gas-gangrene antitoxin or by *Clostridium sordellii* antitoxin (Rifkin *et al*. 1977). Anaerobic cultures of stools of hamsters with the disease revealed large numbers of *C. difficile* (Bartlett *et al*. 1978a, Larson *et al*. 1978). These organisms produced a toxin *in vitro* that resembled the one found in the feces of hamsters dying with antibiotic-induced enterocolitis (Chang *et al*. 1978a), and this toxin was neutralized by *C. sordellii* antitoxin. After *Clostridium difficile* isolates were determined to be susceptible to vancomycin, it was found that this antibiotic could prevent or delay the onset of the antibiotic-induced disease in hamsters treated with vancomycin as well by the oral route (Browne *et al*. 1977a, Bartlett *et al*. 1977b, Bartlett *et al*. 1978b, Larson *et al*. 1980). Koch's postulates were eventually fulfilled for *Clostridium difficile* in hamsters (Chang *et al*. 1978a, Bartlett 1979 , Bartlett *et al*. 1979b). Finally, passive immunization of hamsters with polyvalent clostridial antitoxin protected hamsters from the enterocolitis induced by clindamycin (Allo *et al*. 1979).

It was next found that *Clostridium difficile* and its cytotoxin were present in the stools of humans with pseudomembranous colitis (PMC) (George *et al*. 1978a, Bartlett *et al*. 1978a). Furthermore, patients with PMC responded to treatment with oral vancomycin (Tedesco *et al*. 1978a, Fekety *et al*. 1980, Silva *et al*. 1980a, Silva *et al*. 1981), which appeared to decrease production of the cytotoxin (Taylor *et al*. 1980).

Clostridium difficile is now known to produce at least two toxins, both of which may have a role in antibiotic-induced enterocolitis (Taylor *et al*. 1981, Banno *et al*. 1981, Sullivan *et al*. 1982). The first one detected, now called toxin B, is primarily a cytotoxin (Taylor *et al*. 1979). The cells used to detect its characteristic cytopathic effect are not killed (Donta and Shaffer, 1980) and its mechanism of action is not settled. The other toxin

(toxin A) is lethal and enterotoxic for rodents, but is only weakly cytotoxic. These proteinaceous toxins have been difficult to purify (Sullivan et al. 1982). Consequently, their exact nature and the mechanisms of their cellular action have not been firmly established. There is evidence they alter the function of cell membranes, possibly by an effect upon the guanylate cyclase system (Chang et al. 1979b, Donta and Shaffer, 1980, Thelestam and Bronnegard 1980, Rothman and Brown 1981 Gurwith et al. 1982). Lyerly, Libby, Wilkins and their associates reported it was necessary to immunize hamsters with toxoids prepared from both toxins in order to protect against antibiotic-induced enterocolitis (Libby and Wilkins 1982, Lyerly et al. 1982, Libby et al. 1982).

As will be discussed, it is sometimes possible to produce antibiotic-induced enterocolitis in guinea pigs, rabbits, and gnotobiotic rats or mice, but the best and most extensively studied model of the disease as it occurs in humans is the one utilizing hamsters.

ANTIBIOTIC-ASSOCIATED ENTEROCOLITIS IN HAMSTERS

Production of the disease in this rodent species requires three factors: first, a susceptible (non-immune) hamster; second, exposure to toxigenic *Clostridium difficile* (the source can be endogenous or exogenous); and third, some factor such as antibiotic therapy that disturbs the normal intestinal flora of the animal, thus permitting overgrowth of *C. difficile* and production of its toxins in quantities sufficient to produce the disease.

Hamsters are normally highly resistant to colonization and infection with *Clostridium difficile* (Larson et al. 1978). Since their resistance is easily overcome by the administration of antibiotics, it is unlikely to be attributable to humoral immunity. Most investigators have utilized 6-8 week old male Golden Syrian hamsters (*Mesocricetus auratus*) weighing about 60-100 gm. Female hamsters are also susceptible. Diet may play a role in susceptibility (Michelich et al. 1981). We have been unable to demonstrate antitoxin to toxin B in the sera of older hamsters (32-36 weeks) or hamsters who have not died after receiving antibiotics (Silva et al. 1980b).

While most investigators have reported Clostridium difficile cannot be isolated from the stools of hamsters freshly received from breeding colonies and untreated with antimicrobials, we have been able to isolate C. difficile from the stools of about 3-5 percent of healthy untreated hamsters (Fekety et al. 1980, Toshniwal et al. 1981). While available methods for culturing stools for C. difficile are not adequate for detection of the organism unless it is present in concentrations greater than about 100 CFU/ml, most investigators believe that antibiotic-treated hamsters with enteritis usually have acquired the organism from environmental sources, or human contacts, or as a result of intentional colonization (O'Connor et al. 1981, Toshniwal et al. 1981, Larson et al. 1980 , Wilson et al. 1981). When untreated hamsters were given toxigenic Clostridium difficile in large numbers (>10,000 CFU) orally they remained well, while only a few organisms were required to colonize and kill antibiotic-treated hamsters (Larson et al. 1978, Larson 1980). It appears that one or more members of the normal intestinal flora of hamsters are important in suppressing or resisting colonization and overgrowth by Clostridium difficile (Rolfe and Finegold 1980).The identity of the protective organisms is not known. Antibiotic-treated hamsters were protected from enterocolitis when they were administered feces from normal hamsters via the orogastric route and by enema (Wilson et al. 1981). Considering these facts, it is not surprising that concerns have been raised about the variability and reproducibility of the hamster model of enterocolitis.

Many investigators, including ourselves, have been unable to produce the disease uniformly by administering antibiotics to hamsters. While the response is unpredictable, we believe the variability is attributable to the occasional absence of toxigenic Clostridium difficile isolates in the environment or contacts of antibiotic-challenged hamsters. Thus, if hamsters are not exposed to the organism, they cannot develop the disease. As mentioned, Larson et al. (1978) showed that vancomycin-treated hamsters could be colonized and killed by as few as 1-2 CFU of Clostridium difficile, while untreated animals resisted colonization even when given as many as 10,000 CFU of Clostridium difficile. Also, it should be recognized that some isolates of Clostridium difficile are either non-toxigenic or only weakly toxigenic (Rolfe and Finegold1980 Taylor,Bartlett1979, Banno et al. 1981), and that acquisition of such organisms might protect against acquisition of toxigenic organisms and the disease (see chapter 8).

Because hamsters are cannibalistic as well as coprophagic, the antibiotic-induced disease may occur with high frequency even if only a few animals in a cage initially carry the organism or contact it in their environment. Indeed, when animals are housed individually, or in plastic isolators, or in laminar air flow cage racks in order to prevent transmission of the organism from one hamster to another, the disease occurs much less uniformly (Larson 1980 , Toshniwal et al. 1981). Under these conditions it may be necessary to intentionally colonize hamsters with C. difficile in order to produce enterocolitis following administration of antibiotics (Larson et al. 1980). In fact, this may be the most reliable way to produce the disease in hamsters.

The hamster model of clindamycin-induced enterocolitis has been studied extensively. Clindamycin is capable of inducing enterocolitis even when small amounts (10-100 mgm/kg) are given. It can be given perorally, subcutaneously, intramuscularly, intraperitoneally, or topically (Lusk et al. 1978, Fekety et al. 1979, Feingold et al. 1979). Attack rates of 100 percent with clindamycin are common, especially after the hamster's environment becomes heavily contaminated with C. difficile. The animals develop profuse watery diarrhea within about 5 to 7 days of challenge with antibiotics. They soon become dehydrated, ataxic and lethargic, develop ruffled fur and brown-stained paws and tail ("wet tail" syndrome), and die. Both Clostridium difficile and its toxins are demonstrable in the stools or cecal contents of hamsters with the disease.

Post-mortem examination reveals a cecum that is enlarged, distended with watery stool, edematous, congested, and hemorrhagic. Light microscopy reveals necrosis, hemorrhage, and acute inflammation of the mucosal epithelium. A thin pseudomembrane consisting of dead and dying epithelial and inflammatory cells enmeshed in fibrin and mucus can often be detected in involved areas, but grossly visible pseudomembranes similar to those seen in humans are not found in hamsters. The cecum is the primary target organ in the hamster, but the distal ileum and colon of hamsters may show inflammatory changes microscopically. The lungs, liver, and kidneys may be hemorrhagic. The characteristic pathologic findings in the intestines of the hamster are commonly referred to as typhlitis, ileocecitis, or enterocolitis.

Other antibiotics capable of inducing this disease when given to hamsters by various routes of administration include lincomycin, erythromycin, penicillin G, ampicillin, cephalothin, cefazolin, cephaloridine, cefamandole, cefoxitin, cefotaxime, moxalactam, chloramphenicol, tetracycline, trimethoprim-sulfamethoxazole, gentamicin, tobramycin, rifampin, metronidazole, tetracycline, and vancomycin (Chang et al. 1978a, Lusk et al. 1978, Bartlett et al. 1978c, Fekety et al. 1979, Toshniwal et al. 1979, Ebright et al. 1981). C. difficile is responsible in all cases. The disease may also occur spontaneously (Rehg and Lu. 1982) or following administration of cancer chemotherapeutic agents (Cudmore et al. 1980). Certain antimicrobials such as chloramphenicol, tetracycline and metronidazole are poor inducers of the disease in hamsters, but with proper conditions of dosing and route of administration even they can be made to trigger it (Fekety et al. 1979). In general, the disease pattern is similar with all these antibiotics, but its onset may be delayed or reduced in frequency depending upon the specific antibiotic, the dose and route of administration, or the antimicrobial susceptibility pattern of the organisms prevalent in the hamster quarters when antibiotics are given. We were unable to induce enterocolitis in hamsters with rifampin until resistant isolates of C. difficile appeared in the hamster quarters.

When antibiotics are given repeatedly and at frequent intervals to hamsters, in some instances the disease onset is delayed until the drugs are discontinued, probably because the prevalent Clostridium difficile strains are susceptible to them. This is often the case with vancomycin (Browne et al. 1977a, Fekety et al. 1979). In other cases, such as with rifampin, where the disease appeared despite continued therapy with a presumably active antimicrobial, a resistant organism may have been selected. With ampicillin and other beta-lactam antibiotics (penicillins or cephalosporins), susceptible strains of C. difficile emerged during therapy and caused cecitis despite continued therapy (Fekety et al. 1979 Rolfe and Finegold 1983). The likely explanation for this paradox is that intestinal beta-lactamases and cephalosporinases were induced by the surviving intestinal flora, with subsequent inactivation of the antibiotic, thus permitting susceptible organisms to multiply and exert their pathogenicity. Clostridium difficile is highly susceptible in vitro to metronidazole, vancomycin, and ampicillin, but we have been able to induce the disease in hamsters with each of these antimicrobials.

Vancomycin and metronidazole have been used successfully to treat PMC in humans, but ampicillin is a frequent co-factor in production of Clostridium difficile colitis in humans and is not used in treatment (Bartlett 1979 , Bartlett et al. 1978c, Burdon et al. 1979, Fekety et al. 1979, Fekety et al. 1981b Dzink and Bartlett, 1980).

When hamsters were given a cecitis-inducing dose of clindamycin or a cephalosporin along with oral vancomycin (3 mg/day), they remained well so long as vancomycin was continued, only to develop cecitis a few days after its discontinuation. While vancomycin can prevent colonization with Clostridium difficile so long as it is given, the predisposing conditions within the gut flora induced by antibiotics are not corrected by vancomycin. These important predisposing abnormalities may persist for many weeks (Browne et al. 1977a). Thus, vancomycin itself is a potent predisposing factor in the hamster. This fact suggests that the important organisms that compete with C. difficile in the intestines are susceptible to vancomycin. When vancomycin alone was given perorally to hamsters exposed to Clostridium difficile, they develop cecitis and died a few days after the drug was discontinued. Similarly, if clindamycin-treated hamsters that developed diarrhea were treated promptly and daily with oral vancomycin, the illness resolved, and the animals recovered, only to die with cecitis once the vancomycin was discontinued. Only a few CFU of Clostridium difficile are needed to infect and kill a vancomycin treated hamster (Larson et al. 1978). Not surprisingly, hamsters do not develop the disease if they are protected from environmental and human sources of Clostridium difficile (Larson 1980 , Toshniwal et al. 1981). Vancomycin given parenterally (intraperitoneally or subcutaneously) to hamsters is neither likely to induce cecitis nor as reliably protective against Clostridium difficile colitis as is vancomycin given orally (Browne et al.1977a,).

Metronidazole is useful in treating pseudomembranous colitis in humans (Johnson et al. 1981). However, when metronidazole was given perorally to hamsters for brief periods, many of them died of Clostridium difficile colitis within a few days. This effect was dose-dependent and not as predictable as with vancomycin (Fekety et al. 1979).

Bacitracin is inhibitory for Clostridium difficile, but not at concentrations as low as with vancomycin or metronidazole (Fekety et al. 1979). Bacitracin has not been reported to induce the disease in hamsters or humans, and it has been used in treatment of humans with antibiotic-associated colitis (Tedesco 1980, Bartlett et al. 1978 c).

Cholestyramine, an anion exchange resin, has been used successfully in treatment of mild cases of pseudomembranous colitis in humans, probably because of its ability to bind the toxin(s) of Clostridium difficile (Kreutzer, Milligan 1978 Taylor and Bartlett 1980). When given perorally to clindamycin-treated hamsters, cholestyramine delayed deaths due to cecitis by 24-48 hours, but did not prevent death (R. Browne, J. Silva, R. Fekety, unpublished paper).

Many C. difficile isolates are susceptible to cephalosporins (Fekety et al. 1979). Orally-administered cephalosporins (such as cephalexin) can prevent clindamycin-induced Clostridium difficile colitis in hamsters for brief periods (Ebright et al. 1981), but their protective effects are limited by emergence of resistant Clostridium difficile isolates or by the induction of cephalosporinases by surviving intestinal organisms (Rolfe and Finegold 1983). When given orally, poorly-absorbed cephalosporins (such as cephalothin) are more effective in temporarily preventing colitis than are well-absorbed derivatives such as cephalexin (Ebright et al. 1981), probably because stool antibiotic concentrations are higher when absorption is poor.

GUINEA PIGS AND ANTIBOTIC-INDUCED ENTEROCOLITIS

When guinea pigs are given lincomycin, clindamycin, or certain other antibiotics, they sometimes develop colitis in which Clostridium difficile and its toxin are implicated. As compared with hamsters, the response in guinea pigs is highly unpredictable (Rehg 1980 , Rehg et al. 1980 , Rothman 1981 Lee and Thomsen, 1982). Factors responsible for the variable induction of antibiotic-induced colitis in these rodents, such as strain variation, dietary and seasonal effects, and resistance to colonization with *Clostridium difficile* have not been studied extensively. Rothman (1981) documented Gram-negative bacteremia in guinea pigs dying with penicillin-induced *Clostridium difficile* colitis. Treatment with oral vancomycin did not reduce the bacteremia. Brophy and Knoop (1982) demonstrated an association between intestinal overgrowth with toxigenic *Bacillus pumilus* and clindamycin-associated enterocolitis in guinea pigs. The toxin produced by this organism was not neutralized by *Clostridium difficile* or *C. sordellii* antitoxin, or by other clostridial antisera.

MICE AND ANTIBIOTIC DIARRHEA

While diarrhea associated with antibiotics has been reported to occur in mice, these rodents seem uniquely resistant to the effects of *Clostridium difficile* toxins present in their intestines (Dabard *et al*. 1979). Even when germ-free mice were colonized with *Clostridium difficile* and large amounts of toxin were produced, the animals rarely died, although they did develop diarrhea and intestinal inflammation. When mice mono-associated with *C. difficile* were given oral vancomycin, spores of the organism became detectable and persisted in stools (Onderdonk *et al*. 1980), even though vegetative forms of the organism as well as toxin production declined markedly.

PSEUDOMEMBRANOUS COLITIS IN RATS

C. difficile colonization caused diarrhea and decreased the cecal size of gnotobiotic rats (Gustafsson *et al*. 1970). In recent studies, germ-free rats were mono-associated with either a toxigenic strain of *C. difficile* or a variant strain producing only very small amounts of toxin (Czuprynski *et al*. 1983). Colonization with the toxigenic strain was followed by death of 17 percent of the animals. Large numbers of the organism were present throughout the gastrointestinal tracts of rats dying with diarrhea, but the largest numbers were present in the ceca and colon (10^{10} to 10^{11} CFU/gm). The organism was also isolated from spleens, liver, and kidneys of sacrificed animals. When moribund animals were sacrificed five days after monoassociation, they were found to have toxin-positive cecal filtrates, severe ileitis, ulcerative pseudomembranous colitis, hepatitis, and interstitial pneumonitis. Rats mono-associated with the strain that was a poor toxin producer developed intestinal colonization, but did not have any manifestations of disease. Rats surviving colonization with the toxigenic strain were found to have high titers of neutralizing serum antibody to cytotoxin (1:1,024), while comparable germ-free or conventional rats had no detectable neutralizing antibody in their serum.

ANTIBIOTIC-ASSOCIATED COLITIS IN RABBITS

Rabbits given clindamycin by nasogastric tube (15 mg/kg per day) sometimes developed diarrhea and died. The model seems highly unpredictable, and most antibiotic-treated rabbits do not develop this complication. The illness could be prevented by the co-administration of vancomycin (Katz *et al*. 1978). La Mont and associates (1979) presented evidence that antibiotic-induced enterocolitis in these rabbits was caused by a toxin similar to the iota toxin produced by *Clostridium perfringens* type E, which is cytotoxic for HeLa cells. The toxin caused severe necrosis of rabbit rectal epithelium and was lethal for mice. Evidence was presented recently (Borriello, Carman, 1983) that clindamycin-associated diarrhea as well as spontaneous diarrhea occurring on rabbit farms in Europe and North America was caused by *Clostridium spiroforme*. This helically coiled spore-forming anaerobe was isolated from the intestines of all their rabbits with diarrhea, but rarely from healthy controls. Neither *C. perfringens* type E nor *C. difficile* were isolated from any of the diseased animals. All diseased animals had an iota-like toxin in their cecal contents that was neutralized by *Clostridium perfringens* type E antitoxin. Furthermore, isolates of *C. spiroforme* produced a similar toxin *in vitro*. They also indicated that this organism can induce disease in guinea pigs that have been treated with clindamycin (R.J. Carman, unpublished data). The possible role of this organism in other animal and human diseases deserves further study. Clostridium difficile colitis occurring in a rabbit treated with penicillin and ampicillin for Pasteurellosis has been reported (Rehg and Lu, 1981). Rehg and Pakes (1982) indicated that either Clostridium difficile toxin or C. perfringens iota toxin could induce experimental lincomycin-associated colitis in rabbits.

Dabard and associates (1979) reported that Clostridium difficile, C. perfringens and C. tertium were present together in the stools of young hares with diarrhea, but were rarely encountered in the feces of healthy young hares. When axenic young hares were intentionally colonized with one of these organisms, only animals colonized with Clostridium difficile developed disease. It appeared the numbers of Clostridium difficile had to exceed 10^8/gm of fresh feces for lesions or symptoms to develop. The other species of Clostridia were not pathogenic alone or together, but each appeared to markedly enhance the overgrowth and pathogenicity of Clostridium difficile by some unknown synergistic mechanism. When all three clostridial species were given to conventional young rats, mice, or rabbits, they did not exert any pathogenic role.

CHINCHILLA MODELS OF ENTEROCOLITIS INDUCED BY ANTIBIOTICS

The occurrence of pseudomembranous enterocolitis in chinchillas in association with intestinal overgrowth of Staphylococcus aureus was reported in 1956 following use of chlortetracycline as a food supplement (Wood et al. 1956). When neomycin and bacitracin were added to the drinking water of these rodents and the chlortetracycline was discontinued, the disease in the colony stopped abruptly even though staphylococci were not eliminated from the stools of all animals. When staphylococcal enterotoxins were given intragastrically to chinchillas, Rhesus monkeys or dogs they produced an enteritis characterized by crypt lengthening and an inflammatory cell infiltrate (Van

Prohaska 1959 , Van Prohaska et al. 1959 , Kent 1966, Kocandrle et al. 1966). The role Clostridium difficile may have played in this outbreak was not determined.

SUMMARY

When antibiotics are administered to hamsters or other rodents, diarrhea or colitis may develop. Some rodents seem more susceptible than others. While mice, rats, rabbits, hares, guinea pigs and chinchillas may develop enterocoltiis occasionally, Golden Syrian hamsters are highly and almost uniformly susceptible. When hamsters are given any one of a wide variety of antibiotics by almost any route of administration, a fatal enterocolitis usually ensues within a week. Overgrowth with toxigenic Clostridium difficile is the cause of the disease in hamsters and also of pseudomembranous colitis following antibiotic use in humans. Alterations in the normal intestinal flora are important factors in the pathogenesis of colitis in hamsters and presumably in humans, since the absence of certain competing organisms appears to permit C. difficile to overgrow and produce its toxins. Prevention of antibiotic-induced overgrowth of C. difficile by administration to hamsters of orally administered antibiotics to which C. difficile is reliably susceptible is markedly effective in suppression of acquisition of C. difficile, and in prevention of the disease. It is apparent the hamster model of enterocolitis has been a key factor in determining the pathogenesis and management of C. difficile colitis in humans.

CHAPTER 12

THE PATHOLOGY OF ANTIBIOTIC-ASSOCIATED COLITIS

A. B. PRICE

INDEX

THE PATHOLOGY OF ANTIBIOTIC-ASSOCIATED COLITIS

ASHLEY. B. PRICE

INTRODUCTION

Although antibiotic associated colitis (AAC) is not synonymous with pseudomembranous colitis (PMC) as defined later, PMC is the obvious starting point for any pathological discussion of the topic.

In the modern era PMC is regarded as an iatrogenic disease associated with administration of antibiotics, but of course it did exist well before antibiotics were discovered (Penner & Bernheim 1939). In that period it was seen mostly as a complication of intestinal surgery (Dixon & Weisman, 1948) and the characteristic membranous lesions could be found throughout the gut. Today antibiotic associated PMC seems to be limited to the large bowel. Furthermore, with the discovery of its aetiology (Bartlett et al 1978a) the morphological descriptions of the classical disease need modification.

PSEUDOMEMBRANOUS COLITIS

However it is simplest to commence with the typical picture (Goulston & McGoven, 1965, Price & Davies, 1977). Because the disease is a mucosal one the surgeon may see no peritoneal abnormality in the event of a patient coming to laparotomy. The affected bowel may be slightly dilated and hyperaemic. Toxic megacolon is a recorded but rare occurrence (Cone & Wetzel, 1982). When the bowel is opened the mucosa is seen to be covered by discrete yellow/white plaques varying in size from a few millimetres to about 2 cms. (Fig. 1). Between these the mucosa may look only

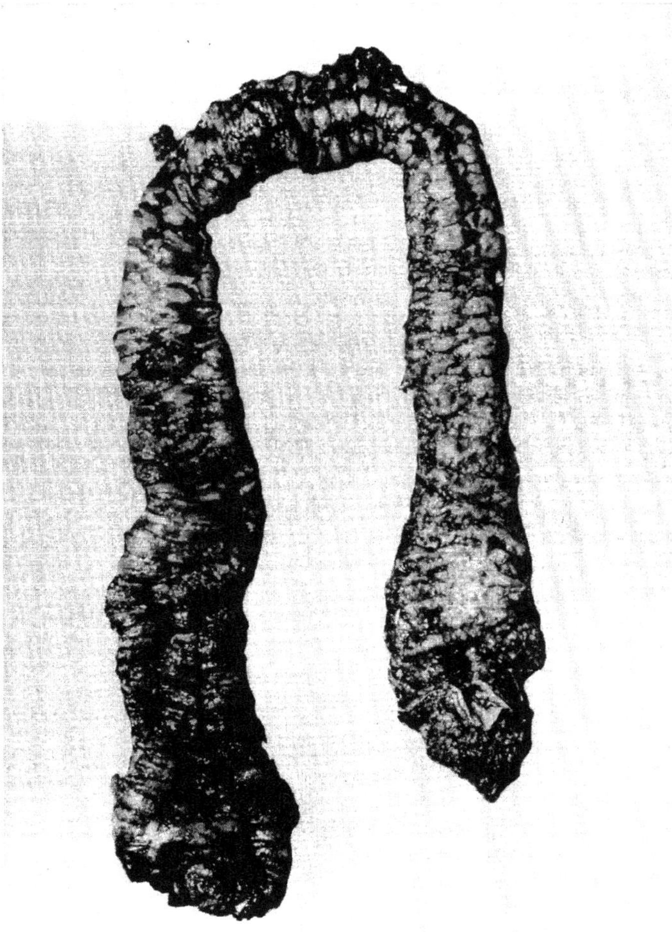

Fig. 1. A total colectomy specimen showing the classical yellow membranes of pseudomembranous colitis throughout the colon.

congested. Once the plaques enlarge much over 2 cms they tend to become confluent and the bowel surface appears covered by varying lengths of shaggy yellowish membrane representing the necrotic mucosa. (Fig. 2).

The factors controlling the distribution and growth of the lesions are not known but in patients whose disease is severe enough to come to surgery, it is customary to find the major length of the large bowel involved. It is clear

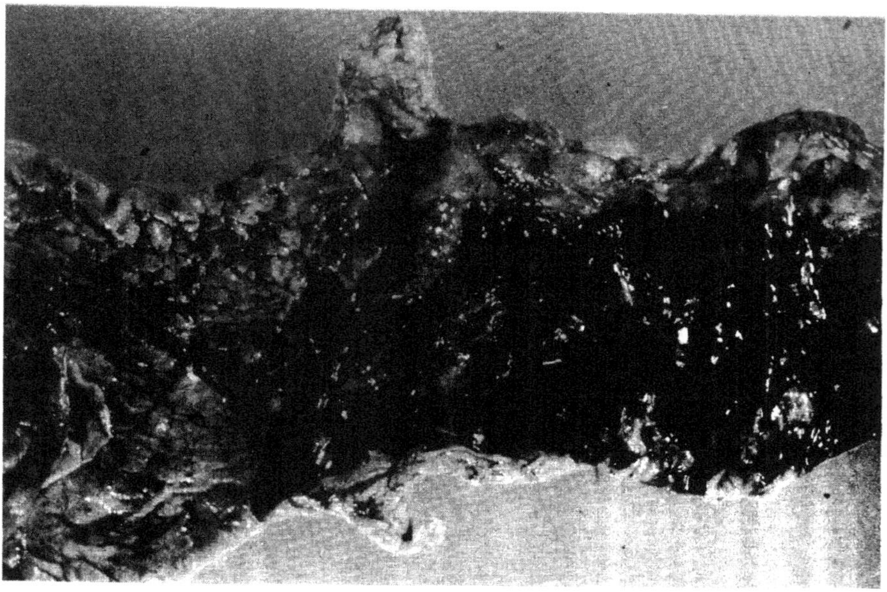

Fig. 2. In this colectomy specimen the plaques have coalesced to give complete mucosal necrosis and yellow necrotic slough can be peeled off the surface.

however from colonoscopic studies that at some stage plaques are limited to one or other segment of the bowel and that the rectum and sigmoid regions may be spared though not necessarily normal. While Tedesco et al (1982) showed plaques in the sigmoid colon and rectum of 91% of patients in a prospective series, Seppala et al (1980) claimed only 31% had sigmoid or rectal lesions, the remainder requiring colonoscopy for their demonstration. The true incidence of recto-sigmoid involvement is important clinically as an examining physician must be aware that an absence of rectal lesions does not exclude the disease.

The histological picture corresponding to the discrete plaques is equally characteristic (Price & Davies, 1977). Each plaque represents a small focus of disrupted crypts (Fig. 3). The bases often survive while the superficial

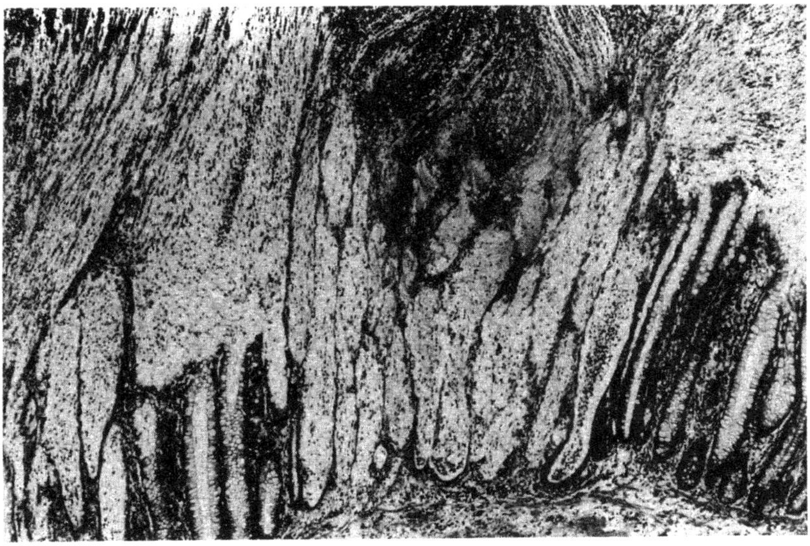

Fig. 3. Typical pseudomembranous colitis is seen in this microphotograph. In the centre is a group of disrupted crypts with a surface coverin of inflammatory debris. Uninvolved mucosa is seen to each side with a second plaque appearing at the left margin. (H. E. x 55).

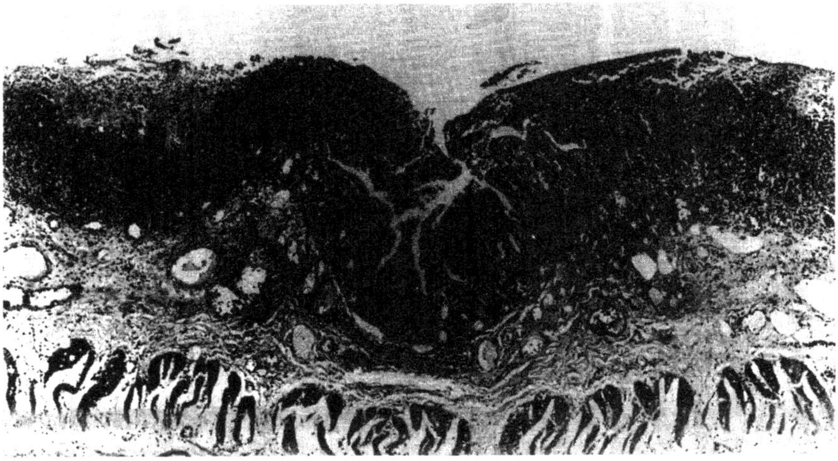

Fig. 4 The type III lesion of nearly complete mucosal necrosis corresponding to the macroscopic features in Fig. 2. (H. E. x 45).

two-thirds are dilated and filled with degenerating absorptive and goblet cells, liberated mucus, fibrin and acute inflammatory cells. All these coalesce to form the yellow plaque visible on the mucosal surface. Although the cellular components of the crypt are lost, their ghost outlines remain. The mucosa between such foci will be either normal, show slight oedema or small

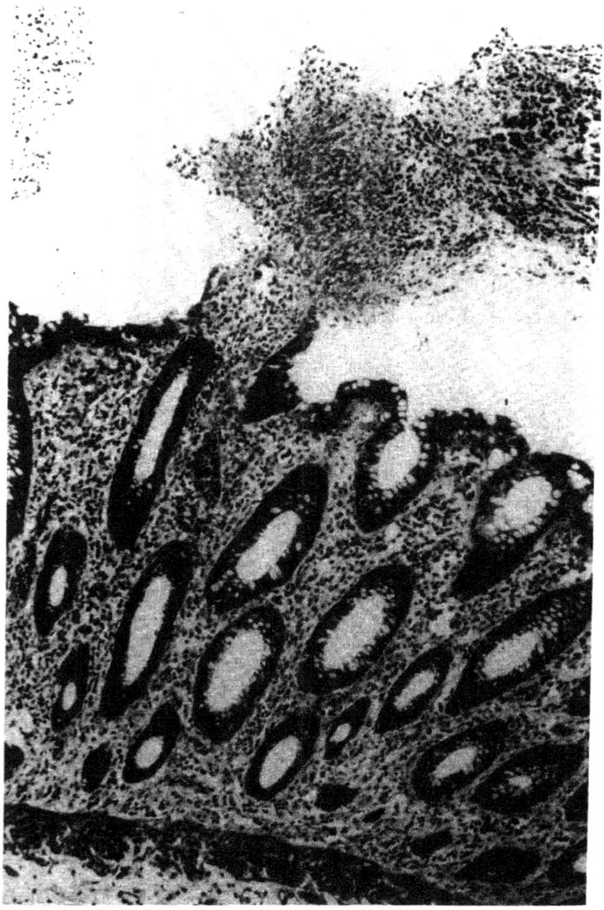

Fig. 5. An intercryptal "summit-lseion" in a virtually normal mucosa. The earliest phase from which pseudomembranous colitis can be diagnosed (H.E. x 105).

clusters of polymorphs involving individual crypts and surface epithelium.

As the lesions enlarge the crypt destruction becomes more complete so that a stage is reached when a layer of inflammatory slough rests on the muscularis mucosae (Fig. 4). At the point of full thickness mucosal necrosis the features are no longer diagnostic and merge with other conditions which have a stage of complete mucosal necrosis, e.g. ischaemia, radiation damage. At this stage a biopsy as well as the surgical specimen may be difficult to interpret.

In the early stages of the development of the typical lesion and prior to recognisable macroscopic lesions one may find tiny superficial intercryptal erosions. Between two crypts the surface epithelium is destroyed and replaced by a wisp of fibrin and acute inflammatory cells (Fig. 5). This "summit-lesion" (Price & Davies, 1977) represents the earliest stage at which a confident morphological diagnosis can be made. The adjacent mucosa must show no more than oedema, focal clusters of polymorphs and perhaps some loss of mucus in adjacent crypts. This is because superficial erosions of the mucosa seem a part of many forms of mucosal damage but are then accompanied by changes appropriate to the condition in question (Fig. 6). Failure to appreciate this may account for lesions of PMC being described in unusual clinical settings (Goulston & McGovern, 1980).

The three patterns, the summit lesion, the focal crypt lesion and the stage of confluent mucosal necrosis represent three steps in the evolution of the pathology, designated types I, II and III by Price & Davies, 1977. Apart from the rare documentation of cases of PMC in which toxic megacolon supervenes (Cone & Wetzel, 1982) the significant histological changes remain confined to the mucosa. The submucosa is oedematous and contains scattered inflammatory cells. Capillary microthrombi are a variable feature and prior to the discovery of the role of _Clostridium difficile_ were at one time felt to be of prime aetiological importance (Whitehead, 1971). It is still possible that the toxins of Clostridium difficile may mediate mucosal damage via a vascular mechanism.

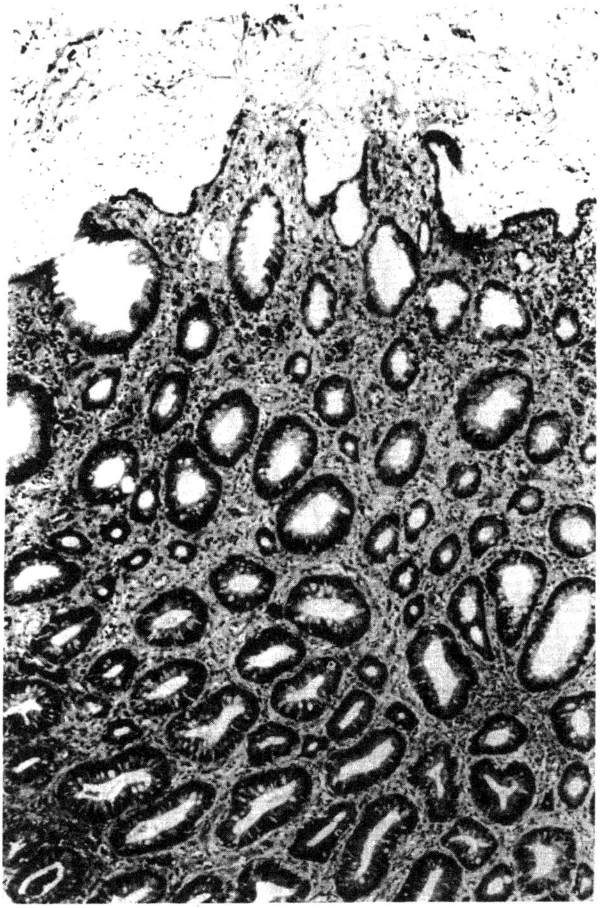

Fig. 6. This shows a tubular adenoma but with surface erosions much like the summit lesion of Fig. 5. This emphasises the importance of interpreting the surface lesion in relation to any adjacent pathology. In this case the lesions were probably the result of surface trauma (H.E. x 30).

BIOPSY DIAGNOSIS

Now that the aetiology of PMC is established and the efficacy of treatment with Vancomycin or Metranidazole has been demonstrated (Tedesco et al. 1978, Pashby et al. 1979) no case should come to surgery. A rapid diagnosis is required in cases with severe colitis and the diagnosis is one of the few justifiable indications for requesting a rapid frozen section on a rectal biopsy specimen. The view at sigmoidoscopy is often diagnostic and the pathologist may see the plaques macroscopically on the surface of the biopsy. Frozen section forms the quickest means of diagnosis as toxin studies and culture require overnight delays. Even though plaques, as described earlier, are not always present in the rectum and because colonoscopy is contra-indicated in patients with acute severe colitis, a rectal

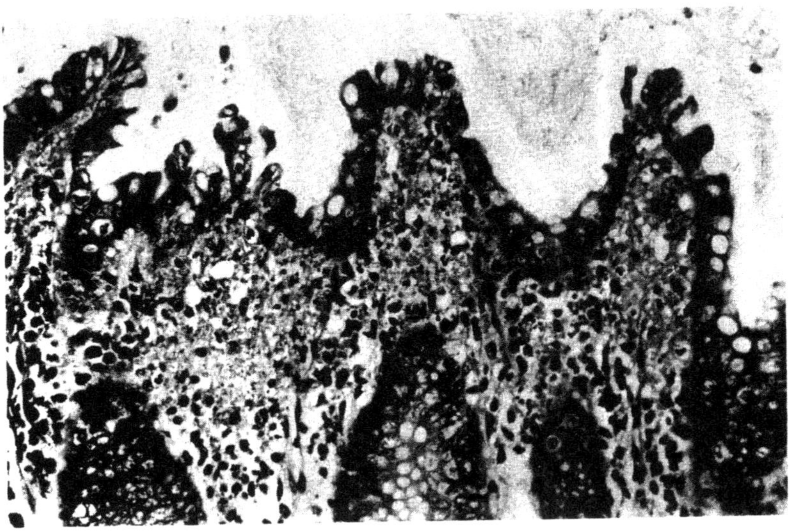

Fig. 7. A biopsy from a patient who was toxin positive but had no pseudomembranes. It shows a crenated and tufted epithelial surface beneath which is a mild acute inflammatory infiltrate (H.E. x 150).

biopsy is always worthwhile. The tiny T.I lesions may not be visible to the naked-eye but the mucosa can still show helpful histological changes in the absence of typical lesions (Fig. 7). Observations on biopsy material from patients with diarrhoea who are toxin positive but with no proven rectal plaques show that the majority are still abnormal. A pattern frequently seen is of an oedematous mucosa, congested, with small clusters of subepithelial polymorphs, some infiltrating the crypts or surface. The epithelium of the latter is often crenated formed by small tufts of epithelial cells (Price & Day, 1981). This picture is qualitatively similar to that seen in other bacterial diarrhoeas (Price et al, 1979a) and while probably not diagnostic does warrant a prompt to the clinician to consider antibiotic-associated disease as part of the differential diagnosis.

TERMINOLOGY

Any discussion of PMC is incomplete without a consideration of the definitions of disease for since the use of toxin assays as a diagnostic tool the terminology has become confusing. PMC as described here is a morphological diagnosis and to be distinguished from antibiotic-associated colitis, AAC, (patients with diarrhoea following a course of antibiotics and biopsy evidence of colitis but no pseudomembranes) and antibiotic-associated diarrhoea, AAD, (patients with diarrhoea, a history of recent antibiotics but normal biopsies). Within these definitions toxin is seen in 6% of patients with AAD, 38% with AAC but 97% of those with PMC (Bartlett et al, 1978d). Clostridium difficile and its toxin therefore seem to define a group of patients with AAD who are most at risk of developing PMC. The factors determining the balance between AAD, AAC and PMC in terms of Clostridium difficile and its toxin still remain to be worked out. There is a satistically significant correlation between a high toxin titre and the presence of PMC and between

PMC and the duration of diarrhoea (Burdon et al, 1981) but these correlations do not hold on an individual patient level. To emphasize this Lishman et al. (1981a) reported a group of patients exposed to antibiotics, without diarrhoea, but with toxin titres in the same range as those with diarrhoea. Clearly there is more to be learnt about the inter-relationship of organism, toxin, antibiotics, mucosal pathology and diarrhoea. Indeed an atypical transient right sided colitis following ampicillin has been described that may be unrelated to Clostridium difficile and PMC (Sakurai et al, 1979). As yet however no such case has come to surgery and a full pathological examination.

COMPARATIVE PATHOLOGY

Enterocolitis following antibiotics and/or exposure to Clostridium difficile occurs in many animals (see Chapter II). The observations by Small (1968) that Lincomycin produced a fatal enterocolitis in hamsters has meant that most comparative work has been carried out in this animal. In micro-biological and epidemiological terms it has been excellent but it is a less satisfactory model from the morphological viewpoint though the one with the best documented pathology. Antibiotic-induced Clostridium difficile associated disease in the hamster remains limited to the caecum and is not colonic as in the human. Two basic patterns are described (Price et al, 1979b), in one there is gross caecal distension with widespread haemorrhage, in the second the caecum may remain of normal size but the mocosa has a thickened velvet texture often with punctate haemorrhages. The histological pattern corresponding to the distended haemorrhagic caecum is one of gross intra-mucosal haemorrhage (Fig. 8). The thickened caecum on histological examination shows elongated crypts with marked "tufting" of the intercrypt surface epithelium (Fig. 9). These heaped up epithelial cells show

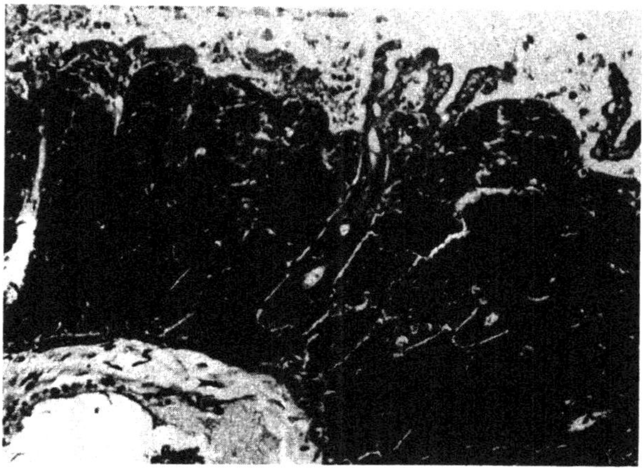

Fig. 8. Gross mucosal haemorrhage in the caecum of a hamster with clindamycin-induced caecitis. (H.E. x 290).

vacuolation and signs of degeneration. A variable degree of inflammation is seen with polymorphs in the lamina propria and infiltrating the surface and crypts. Ulceration is rare (Price et al, 1979b). The surface epithelial changes have been produced by injecting sterile filtrates from Clostridium difficile cultures into the caecum of normal hamsters (Abrams et all, 1980). The resemblance of the above lesions to the classical picture of human PMC is clearly limited. It is of interest to note that in animals challenged with non-pathogenic Clostridium difficile (Borriello, Price and Barclay, unpublished data), minor epithelial changes are found in the caecum (Fig. 10) much like those seen in human biopsy material from patients with diarrhoea, toxin the stool but no proven pseudomembranes (Fig. 7).

The literature descriptions of antibiotic-indiced colitis in guinea pigs, hares, rabbits, rats and mice have limited pathological data (Lowe et al, Dabard et al, 1979, La Mont et al 1979, Czuprynski et al, 1983, Onderdonk et al, 1980). Often the presence of ulceration and ulcer slough is overenthusiastically equated with pseudomembrane. However in some

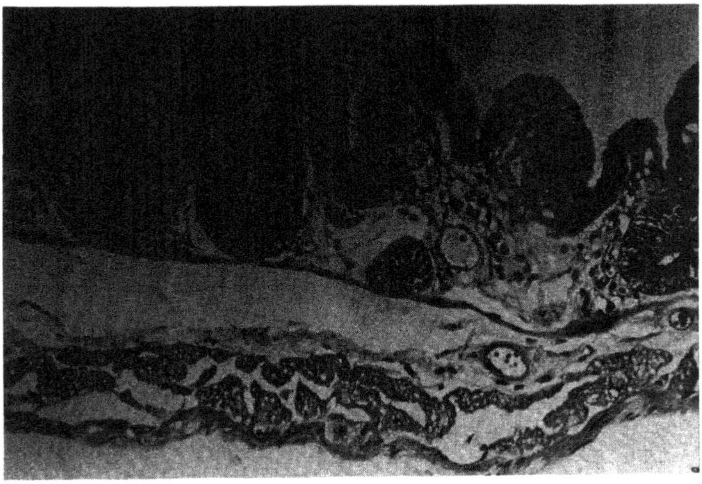

Fig. 9. A & B. The thickened caecal mucosa seen in 9B (below) of the proliferative response in antibiotic-induced caecitis is well seen and in marked contrast to a normal caecum in 9A (above) for comparison (H.E. x 225).

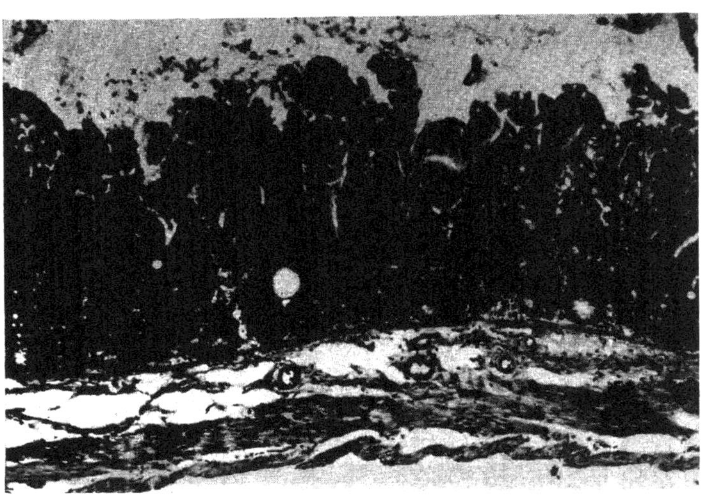

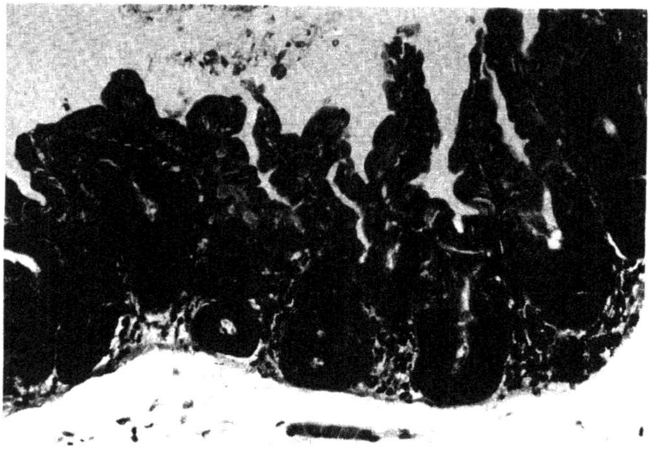

Fig. 10. The minor changes in the epithelial surface from a hamster challenged with clindamycin and a non-pathogenic strain of *Clostridium difficile*. There is some resemblance to Fig. 7. (H.E. x 290).

gnotobiotic experimental models colonic lesions are present which at least are more akin to the diseae distribution in man than the purely caecal disease of the hamster (Czuprynski *et al*, 1983). Because the human disease is so characteristic and specific it is difficult to find an exact animal equivalent. This of course may not be possible for reasons either unique to the human colonic structure or until more is known about the precise pathogenesis of the pseudomembranous lesion.

FUTURE AIMS

Even though *Clostridium difficile* is now accepted as a cause, if not the only cause of PMC, little is known about the pathogenesis of the unique diagnostic lesions. For the pathologist this remains an intriguing question. When this is answered, questions about the spectrum of pathology seen in response to antibiotics may also be clearer. To this end an improved morphological model must be a high priority.

Concluding remarks - the unanswered questions

Despite the tremendous increase in our understanding of C. difficile mediated gastrointestinal disease made over the last five years a great number of important questions remain unanswered. Although it is known that most antibiotics, and even in some cases non-antimicrobial chemotherapeutic agents, will induce disease, it is not known why some antibiotics have a higher associated risk than others or why the parenterally administered aminoglycosides carry a very low risk. In the majority of cases cessation of the offending antibiotic is sufficient to bring about resolution of symptoms within 10 to 14 days. This raises the possibility that specific treatment directed against C. difficile may occasionally exacerbate the situation over the long term by inducing a series of relapses of which some may progress to pseudomembranous colitis. It appears tha not all adult patients who carry C. difficile progress from antibiotic-associated diarrhoea through antibiotic-associated colitis to pseudomembranous colitis. How could we differentiate those patients who would suffer only a mild self-limiting diarrhoea from those who would develop life threatening disease if left untreated? It would be interesting to know what factors are involved in determining the type of disease a patient will develop. In this respect, it is of interest that people over 60 appear to be more likely to suffer a more severe form of the disease than younger people.

One of the most difficult observations to explain is the apparent asymptomatic carriage in infants, especially as cytotoxin can frequently be detected in the stools, sometimes in very high titres, and it is now evident that the 'enterotoxin' is also frequently present. In addition, strains of *C. difficile* from healthy infants have been shown to be pathogenic in animal models. It is possible that infants lack specific mucosal adhesion sites for *C. difficile*, which may explain the transient nature of the carriage noted in most cases, and that adhesion is in some way an important step in the disease process. It is also possible that toxin binding sites are absent, though this is unlikely, or that they are blocked in some way. It is difficult to explain cases of asymptomatic carriage in adults, especially when toxins can be detected in the faeces. In some cases in both infants and adults, strains of *C. difficile* that are cytotoxigenic *in vitro* are isolated when there is no detectable cytotoxin in the faeces.

It is known for many other enteric pathogens that the ability to associate with gastrointestinal mucosa is important for expression of full pathogenic potential. This has been little studied for *C. difficile* though it has been shown that *C. difficile* can be found intimately associated with the gut mucosa in man (Borriello, 1979) and that it adheres to the mucosal lining of the caecum of hamsters (Borriello, 1983). It is possible that some of the toxigenic but non-pathogenic strains of *C. difficile* are non-adhesive variants. It is also unknown whether or not *C. difficile* is invasive, or why discrete plaques form, frequently only within a certain part of the large bowel during early stages of the disease, considering that the organism and its toxins are presumably distributed throughout the gut. It is true to say that little is known about the pathogenesis of this unique diagnostic lesion.

Although it is fairly certain that components of the normal gut flora are important in preventing colonization by *C. difficile*, the actual combination of components necessary to prevent infection have not been well defined. It is also important to interpret antagonism demonstrated *in vitro* between two different organisms with care. This is highlighted by the fact that antagonism between *C. difficile* and streptococci, noted on culture of a faecal specimen (Malamou-Ladas and Tabaqchali, 1982), was interpreted as indicting that streptococci are important in preventing colonization with *C. difficile* despite the fact that both organisms were present in this patient. To date no work has been done to find a simple indirect marker indicative of the state of resistance to colonization by *C. difficile*. Such a marker would be valuable in allowing identification of 'at risk' patients.

Much is still to be learnt about the nature and mechanisms of action of the two *C. difficile* toxins. Very little is known about the 'enterotoxin' and although there is more information available on the cytotoxin a number of basic questions remain unanswered, such as the identity of both the cell surface structure responsible for binding and the intracellular target for toxin action, the significance of inhibition of the cytopathic effect (CPE) by addition of nucleotides to the test system, the relevance of cGMP stimulation in the disease process, and whether cGMP activation noted in tissue culture is primary or secondary to the observed CPE.

Finally, and most importantly, what is the cause of those cases of antibiotic-associated diarrhoea and colitis for which no aetiological agent can yet be ascribed? Recent work from our laboratory has shown that some cases are due to enterotoxigenic *C. perfringens* (Borriello and Larson, unpublished observations), showing that this organism can cause gut disease other than food-poisoning. It is obvious that other pathogens await discovery.

S.P. Borriello

REFERENCE SECTION

A

Abbott, W.G. and Caughey, D.E. (1982). Reactive arthritis due to Clostridium difficile. New Zealand Medical Journal, 95: 287.

Abeyesundere, R.L. (1982). A ward outbreak of Clostridium difficile enterocolitis. Journal of Infection, 5: 277-282.

Abrams, G.D. and Bishop, J.E. (1966). Effect of the normal microbial flora on the resistance of the small intestine to infection. Journal of Bacteriology, 92: 1604-1608.

Abrams, G.D., Allo, M., Rifkin, G.D., Fekety, R. and Silva, J. (1980). Mucosal damage mediated by clostridial toxin in experimental clindamycin-associated colitis. Gut, 21: 493-499.

Allo, M., Silva, J., Fekety, R., Rifkin, G.D. and Waskin, H. (1979). Prevention of clindamycin-induced colitis in hamsters by Clostridium sordellii antitoxin. Gastroenterology, 76: 351-355.

Alpers, D.H. (1978). The pseudomembranous enterocolitides. In Gastrointestinal Disease eds. Sleisenger, M.H. and Fordtran, J.S. W.B. Saunders Company, Philadelphia. pp. 1715-1730.

Aronsson, B., M. Granstrom, R. Mollby, and C.E. Nord (1982a). Toxin A (enterotoxin) from Clostridium difficile in antibiotic-associated colitis. The Lancet, ii: 1279.

Aronsson, B., Möllby, R. and Nord, C.E. (1982b). Clostridium difficile and Antibiotic Associated Diarrhoea in Sweden. Scandinavian Journal of Infectious Diseases (Suppl), 35: 53-58.

Arnon, S.S. (1980). Honey, infant botulism and the sudden infant death syndrome. Western Journal of Medicine, 132: 58-59.

Aswell, J.E., Ehrich, M., Van Tassell, R.L., Tsai, C., Holdeman, L.V. and Wilkins, T.D. (1979). Characterization and comparison of Clostridium difficile and other clostridial toxins. Microbiology-1979: 272-275.

B

Banno, Y., Kobayashi, T., Watanabe, K., Ueno, K. and Nozawa, Y. (1981). Two toxins (D-1 and D-2) of Clostridium difficile causing antibiotic-associated colitis: purification and some characterization. Biochemistry International, 2: 629-635.

Barclay, F.E. and Borriello, S.P. (1982). In vitro inhibition of C. difficile. The European Journal of Chemotherapy and Antibiotics, 2: 155-156.

Barnes, E.M., Impey, C.S. and Cooper, D.M. (1980). Manipulation of the crop and intestinal flora of the newly hatched chick. American Journal of Clinical Nutrition 33: 2426-2433.

Bartlett, J. (1979). Antibiotic-associated pseudomembranous colitis. Reviews of Infectious Diseases 1: 530-539.

Bartlett, J.G. (1980). Experimental studies of antibiotic-associated colitis. Scandinavian Journal of Infectious Diseases, (Suppl.), 22: 11-15.

Bartlett, J. (1981a). Clostridium difficile and inflammatory bowel disease. Gastroenterology, 80: 863-865.

Bartlett, J.G. (1981b). Antimicrobial agents implicated in Clostridium difficile toxin-associated diarrhoea or colitis. The Johns Hopkins Medical Journal, 149: 6-9.

Bartlett, J.G. (1982). Clostridium difficile and cytotoxin in feces of patients with antimicrobial agent-associated colitis: Comment on the report by W.L. George et al. Infection, 10: 208.

Bartlett, J.G. (1983). Treatment of antibiotic-associated pseudomembranous colitis. Reviews of Infectious Diseases, (in press).

Bartlett, J.G. and Gorbach, S.L. (1977). Pseudomembranous enterocolitis (Antibiotic-related colitis). Advances in Internal Medicine, 22: 455-476.

Bartlett, J.G., Onderdonk, A.B., Asneros, A.B. and Kasper, D.L. (1977a). Clindamycin associated colitis due to toxin producing species of Clostridium in hamsters. Journal of Infectious Diseases, 136: 701-705.

Bartlett, J.G., Onderdonk, A. and Cisneros, R.L. (1977b). Clindamycin-associated colitis in hamsters: protection with vancomycin. Gastroenterology, 73: 772-776.

Bartlett, J.G., Onderdonk, A.B., Cisneros, R.L. and Kasper, D.L. (1977c). Clindamycin-associated colitis due to a toxin-producing species of Clostridium in hamsters. Journal of Infectious Diseases, 136: 701-705.

Bartlett, J.G., Chang, T-W., Gurwith, M., Gorbach, S.L. and Onderdonk, A.B. (1978a) Antibiotic-associated pseudomembranous colitis due to toxin-producing clostridia. New England Journal of Medicine, 298: 531-534.

Bartlett, J.G., Chang, T-W. and Onderdonk, A.B. (1978b). Comparison of five regimens for treatment of experimental clindamycin-associated colitis. Journal of Infectious Diseases, 138: 81-86.

Bartlett, J.G., Chang, T-W., Moon, N. and Onderdonk, A.B. (1978c). Antibiotic-induced lethal enterocolitis in hamsters: studies with eleven agents and evidence to support the pathogenic role of toxin-producing clostridia. American Journal Veterinary Research, 39: 1525-1530.

Bartlett, J.G., Moon, N., Chang, T-W., Taylor, N., and Onderdonk, A.B. (1978d). Role of Clostridium difficile in antibiotic-associated pseudomembranous colitis. Gastroenterology, 75: 778-782.

Bartlett, J.G., Chang, T-W., Taylor, N.S., and Onderdonk, A.B. (1979a). Colitis induced by Clostridium difficile. Reviews of Infectious Diseases, 1: 370-378.

Bartlett, J.G., Willey, S.H., Chang, T-W., and Lowe, B. (1979b). Cephalosporin-associated pseudomembranous colitis due to Clostridium difficile. Journal of the American Medical Association, 242: 2683-2685.

Bartlett, J.G., Taylor, N.S., Chang, T-W., and Dzink, J. (1980a). Clinical and laboratory observations in Clostridium difficile colitis. American Journal of Clinical Nutrition, 33: 2521-2526.

Bartlett, J.G., Tedesco, F.J., Shull, S., Lowe, B. and Chang, T-W. (1980b). Symptomatic relapse after oral vancomycin therapy of antibiotic-associated pseudomembranous colitis. Gastroenterology, 78: 431-434.

Batts, D.H., Martin, D., Holmes, R., Silva, J., and Fekety, F.R. (1980). Treatment of antibiotic-associated Clostridium difficile diarrhea with oral vancomycin. Journal of Pediatrics, 97: 151-153.

Ben-Zé ev, A., Farmer, S.R. and Penman, S. (1980). Protein synthesis requires cell-surface contact while nuclear events respond to cell shape in anchorage-dependent fibroblasts. Cell, 21: 365-372.

Bolton, R.P., Sherriff, R.J. and Read, A.E. (1980). Clostridium difficile associated diarrhoea: a role in Inflammatory bowel disease. The Lancet, i: 383-384.

Bolton, R.P., Wood, G.M. and Losowsky, M.S. (1981). Acute arthritis associated with Clostridium difficile colitis. British Medical Journal, 283: 1023-1024.

Bone, E., Tamm, A. and Hill, M. (1976). The production of urinary phenols by gut bacteria and their possible role in the causation of range bowel cancer. American Journal of Clinical Nutrition, 29: 1448-1454.

Boquet, P. and Duflot, E. (1982). Tetanus toxin fragment forms channels in lipid vesicles at low pH. Proceedings of the National Academy of Sciences, 79: 7614-7618.

Borriello, S.P. (1978). An evaluated micromethod for the detection of Clostridium difficile enterotoxin. Microbios Letters. 7: 25-28.

Borriello, S.P. (1979). Clostridium difficile and its toxin in the gastrointestinal tract in health and disease. Research and Clinical Forums, 1: 33-35.

Borriello, S.P. (1981a). Clostridial flora of the gastrointestinal tract in health and disease. PhD Thesis. University of London, U.K.

Borriello, S.P. (1981b). Gas-liquid chromatography and Clostridium difficile. The Lancet, ii: 1283.

Borriello, S.P. (1983). Clostridium difficile and gut disease. In Microbes and infections of the gut. ed. C.S. Goodwin. Blackwell Scientific Publications, Oxford. pp. 327-346.

Borriello, S.P., Hudson, M.J. and Hill, M.J. (1978). Investigation of the gastrointestinal bacterial flora. Clinics in Gastroenterology, 7: 329-349.

Borriello, S.P. and Honour, P. (1981). Simplified procedure for the routine isolation of Clostridium difficile from faeces. Journal of Clinical Pathology, 34: 1124-1127.

Borriello, S.P. and Larson, H.E. (1981). Antibiotics and pseudomembranous colitis. Journal of Antimicrobial Chemotherapy, 7: Suppl. A: 53-62.

Borriello, S.P., Larson, H.E., Honour, P. and Barclay, F.E. (1982). Antibiotic-associated diarrhoea and colitis. In Clinical Research Centre Report, Medical Research Council, London. p. 96-98.

Borriello, S.P. and Barclay, F.E. (1983). Clostridium difficile infection - protection by prior colonization with non-pathogenic strains. In Models of Anaerobic Infection, ed. in chief Hill, M.J. Martinus Nijhoff Publishers, The Hague, Boston, London, (In press).

Borriello, S.P., Barclay, F.E. and Welch, A.R. (1983a). Colonization resistance of the gastrointestinal tract - a potential in vitro method for the determination of susceptibility to infection with C. difficile. In Models of Anaerobic Infection ed. in chief Hill, M.J., Martinus Nijhoff Publishers, The Hague, Boston, London (In press).

Borriello, S.P. and Carman, R.J. (1983). Association of iota-like toxin and Clostridium spiroforme with both spontaneous and antibiotic-associated diarrhoea and colitis in rabbits. Journal of Clinical Microbiology, 17: 414-418.

Borriello, S.P., Honour, P., Turner, T., and Barclay, F. (1983b). Household pets as a potential reservoir for Clostridium difficile infection. Journal of Clinical Pathology, 36: 84-87.

Bowden, T.A., Mansberger, A.R. and Lykins, L.E. (1981). Pseudomembranous enterocolitis : mechanism of restoring floral homeostasis. American Surgeon, 47: 178-183.

Brettle, R.P., Poxton, I.R., Murdoch, J.M., Brown, R., Byrne, M.D. and Collee, J.G. (1982). Clostridium difficile in association with sporadic diarrhoea. British Medical Journal, 284: 230-233.

Brewer, G.J. (1980). Calmodulin, zinc, and calcium in cellular and membrane regulation: An interpretive review. American Journal of Hematology, 8: 231-248.

Brook, I. (1980). Isolation of toxin producing Clostridium difficile from two children with oxacillin-and dicloxacillin-associated diarrhoea. Pediatrics, 65: 1154-1156.

Brophy, P.F. and Knoop, F.C. (1982). Bacillus pumilus in the induction of clindamycin-associated enterocolitis in guinea pigs. Infection and Immunity, 35: 289-295.

Brown, J.R.D. (1981). Metronidazole and antibiotic-associated colitis. British Medical Journal, 283: 1334.

Browne, R.A., Fekety, R., Silva, J., Boyd, D.I., Work, C.O. and Abrams, G.D. (1977a). The protective effect of vancomycin on clindamycin-induced colitis in hamsters. Johns Hopkins Medical Journal, 141: 183-192.

Browne, R., Rifkin, G., Silva, J. and Fekety, R. (1977b). Vancomycin suppression of colitis and production of fecal toxin(s) following clindamycin in hamsters. 17th International Science Conference, Antimicrobial Agents and Chemotherapy, Abstract 200.

Bruce, D., Ritchie, C., Jennings, L.C., Lynn, K.L., Bailey, R.R. and Cook, H.B. (1982). Clostridium difficile-associated colitis: cross infection in predisposed patients with renal failure. New Zealand Medical Journal, 95: 265-267.

Burdon, D.W. (1982). Clostridium difficile: the epidemiology and prevention of hospital-acquired infection. Infection, 10: 203-204.

Burdon, D.W., Brown, J.D., Youngs, D.J., Arabi, Y., Shinagawa, N., Alexander-Williams, J. and Keighley, M.R.B. (1979). Antibiotic susceptibility of Clostridium difficile. Journal of Antimicrobial Chemotherapy, 5: 307-310.

Burdon, D.W., Keighley, M.R.B., Allan, R.N. and George, R.H. (1980). Clostridial toxin in inflammatory bowel disease. The Lancet, i: 1421.

Burdon, D.W., George, R.H., Mogg, G.A.G., Arabi, Y., Thompson, H., Johnson, M., Alexander-Williams, J. and Keighley, M.R.B. (1981). Faecal toxin and severity of antibiotic-associated pseudomembranous colitis. Journal of Clinical Pathology, 34: 548-551.

Buts, J.P., Weber, A.M., Roy, C.C. and Morin, C.L. (1977). Pseudomembranous enterocolitis in childhood. Gastroenterology, 173: 823-827.

C

Cashore, W.J., Lauermann, P.G., Stonestreet, B.S. and Oh, W. (1981). Clostridia colonisation and clostridial toxin in neonatal enterocolitis. Journal of Pediatrics, 98: 308-311.

Cato, E.P., Hash, D.E., Holdeman, L.V. and Moore, W.E.C. (1982). Electrophoretic study of Clostridium species. Journal of Clinical Microbiology, 15: 688-702.

Chang, T-W., Bartlett, J.G., Gorbach, S.L. and Onderdonk, A.B. (1978a). Clindamycin-induced enterocolitis in hamsters as a model of pseudomembranous colitis in patients. Infection and Immunity, 20: 526-529.

Chang, T., Gorbach, S.L. and Bartlett, J.G. (1978b). Neutralization of Clostridium difficile toxin by Clostridium sordellii antitoxins. Infection and Immunity, 22: 418-422.

Chang, T., Onderdonk, A.B. and Bartlett, J.G. (1978c). Anion-exchange resins in antibiotic-associated colitis. The Lancet, ii: 624-625.

Chang, T-W., Lauermann, M. and Bartlett, J.G. (1979a). Cytotoxicity assay in antibiotic-associated colitis. Journal of Infectious Diseases, 140: 765-770.

Chang, T-W., Lin, P.S., Gorbach, S.L., and Bartlett, J.G. (1979b). Ultrastructural changes in cultured human amnion cells by Clostridium difficile toxin. Infection and Immunity, 23: 795-798.

Chang, T-W., Gorbach, S.L. and Bartlett, J.G. (1980a). Inhibition of binding of Clostridium difficile toxin by steroids. Journal of Infectious Diseases, 142: 113.

Chang, T-W., Gorbach, S.L., Bartlett, J.G. and Saginur, R. (1980b). Bacitracin in antibiotic-associated colitis and diarrhoea caused by Clostridium difficile toxin. Gastroenterology, 78: 1584-1586.

Chang, T-W., Bartlett, J.G. and Taylor, N.S. (1981). Clostridium difficile toxin. Pharmacology and Therapy, 13: 441-452.

Chang, T-W. and Gorbach, S.L. (1982). Rapid Identification of Clostridium difficile by toxin detection. Journal of Clinical Microbiology, 15: 465-467.

Cherry, R.D., Portnoy, D., Jabbari, M., Daly, D.S., Kinnear, D.G. and Goresky, C.A. (1982). Metronidazole: an alternate therapy for antibiotic-associated colitis. Gastroenterology, 82: 849-851.

Cone, J.B., Wetzel, W. (1982). Toxic megacolon secondary to pseudomembranous colitis. Diseases of the Colon and Rectum, 25: 478-482.

Cooperstock, M.S., Steffan, E., Yolken, R. and Onderdonk, A. (1982). Clostridium difficile in normal infants and sudden infant death syndrome: an association with infant formula feeding. Pediatrics, 70: 91-95.

Cudmore, M.A., Silva, J., and Fekety, R. (1980). Clostridial enterocolitis produced by antineoplastic agents in hamsters and humans. In Current Chemotherapy and Infectious Diseases, American Society for Microbiology, pp. 1460-1461.

Cudmore, M.A., Silva, J.H., Fekety, R., Liepman, M.K., and Kim, K-H. (1982). Clostridium difficile colitis associated with cancer chemotherapy. Archives of Internal Medicine, 142: 333-335.

Czuprynski, C.J., Johnson, W.J., Balish, E., and Wilkins, T. (1983). Pseudomembranous colitis in Clostridium difficile-monoassociated rats. Infection and Immunity, 39: 1368-1376.

D

Dabard, J., Dubos, F., Martinet, L., and Ducluzeau, R. (1979). Experimental reproduction of neonatal diarrhoea in young gnotobiotic hares simultaneously associated with Clostridium difficile and other Clostridium strains. Infection and Immunity, 24: 7-11.

Delfini, C., Amici, C., Belardelli, F., Oberholtzer, G. and Sorrentino, M. (1982). Concanavalin A-induced inhibition of abrin and ricin activity parallels with a decrease of the number of toxin-binding uptake-elution cycles. Experimental Cell Research, 142: 427-435.

Dixon, C.F., and Weisman, R.E. (1948). Acute pseudomembranous enteritis or enterocolitis: a complication following intestinal surgery. Surgery Clinics of North America, 28: 999-1023.

Donta, S.T., and Shaffer, S.J. (1980). Effect of Clostridium difficile toxin on tissue cultured cells. Journal of Infectious Diseases, 141: 218-222.

Donta, S.T., Stuppy, M.S., and Myers, M.G. (1981). Neonatal antibiotic-associated colitis. American Journal of Disease of Children, 135: 181-184.

Donta, S.T. and Myers, M.G. (1982). Clostridium difficile toxin in asymptomatic neonates. Journal of Pediatrics, 100: 431-434.

Donta, S.T., Sullivan, N., and Wilkins, T.D. (1982). Differential effects of Clostridium difficile toxins on tissue-cultured cells. Journal of Clinical Microbiology, 15: 1157-1158.

Dorman, S.A., Liggoria, E., Winn, W.C., and Beeken, W.L. (1982). Isolation of Clostridium difficile from patients with inactive Crohn's disease. Gastroenterology, 82: 1348-1351.

Dowell, V.R., and Hawkins, T.M. (1974). Laboratory methods in anaerobic bacteriology, p.1-96. Center for Disease Control, Atlanta, Ga. DHEW Publ No. (CDC) 74-8272.

Dzink, J., and Bartlett, J.G. (1980). In vitro susceptibility of Clostridium difficile isolates from patients with antibiotic-associated diarrhoea or colitis. Antimicrobial Agents and Chemotherapy, 17: 695-698.

E

Ebright, J.R., Fekety, R., Silva, J., and Wilson, K.W. (1981). Evaluation of eight cephalosporins in hamster colitis model. Antimicrobial Agents and Chemotherapy, 19: 980-986.

El Sanousi, S.M., El Azhari, G., and Adlan, A.M. (1978). The inhibition of Clostridium chauvoei by Bacillus cereus metabolites. Australian Veterinary Journal, 54: 455-456.

Elsden, S.R., Hilton, M.G. and Waller, J.M. (1976). The end products of the metabolism of aromatic amino acids by Clostridia. Archives of Microbiology, 107: 283-288.

Erickson, J.E., and Deibel, R.H. (1978). New medium for rapid screening and enumeration of Clostridium perfringens in foods. Applied and Environmental Microbiology, 36: 567-571.

F

Fainstein, V., Bodey, G.P., and Fekety, R. (1981). Relapsing pseudomembranous colitis associated with cancer chemotherapy. Journal of Infectious Diseases, 143: 865.

Fairweather, S.D., Youngs, D., George, R.H., Burdon, D.W. and Keighley, M.R.B. (1980). Arthritis in pseudomembranous colitis associated with an antibody to Clostridium difficile toxin. Journal of the Royal Society of Medicine, 73: 524-525.

Falsen, E., Kaijser, B., Nehls, L., Nygren, B., and Svedhem, A. (1980). Clostridium difficile in relation to enteric bacterial pathogens. Journal of Clinical Microbiology, 12: 297-300.

Feingold, D.S., Chen, W.C., Chou, D-L., and Chang, T-W. (1979). Induction of colitis in hamsters by topical application of antibiotics. Archives of Dermatology, 115: 580-581.

Fekety, R., Silva, J., Toshniwal, R., Allo, M., Armstrong, J., Browne, R., Ebright, J. and Rifkin, G. (1979). Antibiotic-associated colitis: effects of antibiotics on Clostridium difficile and the disease in hamsters. Reviews of Infectious Diseases, 1: 386-396.

Fekety, R., Kim, K-H., Batts, D.H., Browne, R.A., Cudmore, M.A., Silva, J., Toshniwal, R., and Wilson, K.H. (1980). Studies on the epidemiology of antibiotic-associated Clostridium difficile colitis. American Journal of Clinical Nutrition, 33: 2527-2532.

Fekety, R., Kim, K-H., Brown, D., Batts, D.H., Cudmore, M. and Silva, Jr. J. (1981a). Epidemiology of antibiotic-associated colitis: isolation of Clostridium difficile from the hospital environment. American Journal of Medicine, 70: 906-908.

Fekety, R., Silva, J., Armstrong, J., Allo, M., Browne, R., Ebright, J., Lusk, R., Rifkin, G., and Toshniwal, R. (1981b). Treatment of antibiotic-associated enterocolitis with vancomycin. Reviews Infectious Diseases, 3 (Supplement): S273-S281.

Florin, I., and Thelestam, M. (1981). Intoxication of cultured human lung fibroblasts with Clostridium difficile cytotoxin. Infection and Immunity, 33: 67-74.

Florin, I. and Thelestam, M. (1982). Intoxication of human lung fibroblasts with the cytopathogenic toxin from Clostridium difficile. Toxicon, 20: 203-204.

Florin, I. and Thelestam, M. (1983). Internalization of Clostridium difficile cytotoxin into cultured human lung fibroblasts. In Proceedings of FEMS Workshop Symposium on Bacterial Protein Toxins eds. Jeljaszewicz, J. and Alouf, J. Academic Press, London (in press).

Formal, S.B., Abrams, G.D., Schneider, H. and Sprinz, H. (1963). Experimental Shigella infections. VI. Role of the small intestine in an experimental infection in guinea pigs. Journal of Bacteriology, 85: 119-125.

G

George, R.H. (1979). A micromethod for detecting toxins in pseudomembranous colitis. Journal of Clinical Pathology, 32: 303-304.

George, R.H., Symonds, J.M., Dimock, F., Brown, J.D., Arabi, Y., Shinagawa, N., Keighley, M.R.B., Alexander-Williams, J., and Burdon, D.W. (1978a). Identification of Clostridium difficile as a cause of pseudomembranous colitis. British Medical Journal, 1: 695.

George, W.L. (1980). Antimicrobial agent-associated colitis and diarrhea. Western Journal of Medicine, 133: 115-123.

George, W.L., Sutter, V.L., and Finegold, S.M. (1978b). Toxigencity and antimicrobial susceptibility of Clostridium difficile, a cause of antimicrobial agent-associated colitis. Current Microbiology, 1: 55-58.

George, W.L., Sutter, V.L., Goldstein, E.J.C., Ludwig, S.L. and Finegold, S.M. (1978c). Aetiology of antimicrobial-agent-associated colitis. The Lancet, i: 802-803.

George, W.L., Kirby, B.D., Sutter, V.L., and Finegold, S.M. (1979a). Antimicrobial susceptibility of Clostridium difficile. In: Microbiology-1979, Schlessinger D (ed.), American Society for Microbiology, Washington, D.C., pp. 267-271.

George, W.L., Rolfe, R.D., Mulligan, M.E., and Finegold, S.M. (1979b). Infectious diseases 1979 - antimicrobial agent induced colitis: an update. Journal of Infectious Diseases, 140: 266-268.

George, W.L., Sutter, V.L., Citron, D., and Finegold, S.M. (1979c). Selective and differential medium for isolation of Clostridium difficile. Journal of Clinical Microbiology, 9: 214-219.

George, W.L., Volpicelli, N.A., Stiner, D.B., Richman, D.D., Liechty, E.J., Mok, H.Y.I., Rolfe, R.D., and Finegold, S.M. (1979d). Relapse of pseudomembranous colitis after vancomycin therapy. New England Journal of Medicine, 301: 414-415.

George, W.L., Rolfe, R.D., and Finegold, S.M. (1980). Treatment and prevention of antimicrobial agent-induced colitis and diarrhoea. Gastroenterology, 79: 366-372.

George, W.L., Rolfe, R.D., and Finegold, S.M. (1982a). Clostridium difficile and its cytotoxin in feces of patients with antimicrobial agent-associated diarrhea and miscellaneous conditions. Journal of Clinical Microbiology, 15: 1049-1053.

George, W.L., Rolfe, R.D., Harding, G.M., Klein, R., Putnam, C.W., and Finegold, S.M. (1982b). Clostridium difficile and cytotoxin in feces of patients with antimicrobial agent-associated pseudomembranous colitis. Infection, 10: 205-207.

Giugliano, L.G., Mann, G.F. and Drasar, B.S. (1982). Other enterotoxic enteropathies - The use of tissue culture for the detection of clostridial toxins. European Journal of Chemotherapy and Antibiotics, 2: 139-142.

Gotz, V., Romankiewicz, J.A., Moss, J. and Murray, H.W. (1979). Prophylaxis against ampicillin - associated diarrhea with a lactobacillus preparation. American Journal of Hospital Pharmacy, 36: 754-757.

Goulston, S.J.M. and McGovern, V.J. (1965). Pseudomembranous colitis. Gut, 6: 207-212.

Goulston, S.J.M., and McGovern, V.J. (1980). Clinical settings in pseudomembranous colitis. Australian and New Zealand Journal of Medicine, 10: 139-145.

Greenfield, C., Burroughs, A., Szawathowski, M., Bass, N., Noone, P., and Pounder, R. (1981). Is pseudomembranous colitis infectious? The Lancet, i: 371-372.

Griffin, G.E., Heath, J. and Knox, P. (1982). The action of C. difficile cytotoxin is inhibited by specific glycoproteins. Journal of Medical Microbiology, 15: Pxix (Abstract).

Gurian, L., Ward, T.T., and Katon, R.M. (1982). Possible foodborne transmission in a case of pseudomembranous colitis due to Clostridium difficile. Gastroenterology, 83: 465-469.

Gurwith, M.J., Langston, C., and Citron, D.M., (1981). Toxin-producing bacteria in infants. American Journal of Diseases of Children, 135: 1104-1106.

Gurwith, M.J., Langston, C., and Dunsmore, B. (1982). Morphological and functional effects of Clostridium difficile enterotoxin in tissue culture. Canadian Journal of Microbiology, 28: 100-105.

Gustafsson, B.E., Midtvedt, T., and Strandberg, K. (1970). Effects of microbial contamination on the cecum enlargement of germfree rats. Scandinavian Journal of Gastroenterology, 5: 309-314.

H

Hafiz, S., McEntegart, M.G., Morton, R.S., and Waitkins, S.A. (1975). Clostridium difficile in the urogenital tract of males and females. The Lancet, i: 420-421.

Hafiz, S. and Oakley, C.L. (1976). Clostridium difficile : Isolation and characteristics. Journal of Medical Microbiology, 9: 129-136.

Halebian, S., Mulligan, M., Anselmo, C. and Finegold, S.M. (1983). Serologic typing as a tool for epidemiological studies of Clostridium difficile. In Abstracts of the Annual Meeting of the American Society for Microbiology, 1983. American Society for Microbiology, Washington, D.C. Abstract C196, p. 344.

Hall, J. and O'Toole, E. (1935). Intestinal flora in newborn infants with description of a new pathogenic organism, Bacillus difficilis. American Journal of Diseases of Children, 49: 390-402.

Harvie, N., Ellis, S., Mason, D., Allo, N., Rifkin, G., Silva, J. and Fekety, R. (1978). Isolation and purification of a Clostridium difficile toxin that causes colitis in the Syrian hamster. 18th International Science Conference. Antimicrobial Agents and Chemotherapy, Atlanta, Abstract 130.

Hentges, D.J., and Maier, B.R. (1970). Inhibition of Shigella flexneri by the normal intestinal flora. III. Interactions with Bacteroides fragilis strains in vitro. Infection and Immunity, 2: 364-370.

Hickling, P., and Fuller, J. (1979). Penicillamine causing acute colitis. British Medical Journal, ii: 367.

Higaki, M., Honda, T., Takeda, Y., and Miwatani, T. (1981). Detection of Clostridium difficile toxin in suckling mice. FEMS Microbiology Letters 12: 351-353.

Holdeman, L.V., Cato, E.P. and Moore, W.E.C. (1977). Anaerobe laboratory manual, 4th ed. Virginia Polytechnic Institute and State University, Blacksburg, Virginia, U.S.A.

Holst, E., Helin, I. and Mardh, P.A. (1981). Recovery of Clostridium difficile from children. Scandinavian Journal of Infectious Diseases, 13: 41-45.

Howard, J.M., Sullivan, S.N., and Troster, M. (1980). Spontaneous pseudomembranous colitis. British Medical Journal, 281: 356.

Hsu, C-Y. and Wiseman, G.M. (1967). Antibacterial substances from staphylococci. Canadian Journal of Microbiology, 13: 447-455.

Hubert, J., Ionesco, H. and Sebald, M. (1981). Detection de Clostridium difficile par isolement sur milieu minimal sélectif et pas immunofluorescence. Annals Microbiology (Institute Pasteur), 132A: 149-157.

Humphrey, C.D., Condon, C.W., Cantey, J.R., and Pittman, F.E. (1979). Partial purification of a toxin found in hamsters with antibiotic-associated colitis. Gastroenterology, 76: 468-476.

I

Impey, C.S., Mead, G.C. and George, S.M. (1982). Competitive exclusion of salmonellas from the chick caecum using a defined mixture of bacterial isolates from the caecal microflora of an adult bird. Journal of Hygiene, Cambridge, 89: 479-490.

Ionesco, H. (1978). Initiation de la germination des spores de Clostridium difficile par le lysozyme. Comptes rendus Academie des Sciences (Paris), Supplement aux Series D, 287: 659-661.

Ionesco, H. (1980). Transferable tetracycline resistance in Clostridium difficile. Annals of Microbiology, 131: 171-179.

J

Jarvis, W., Nunez-Montiel, O., Thompson, F., Dowell, V., Towns, M., Morris, G., and Hill, E. (1983). Comparison of bacterial isolation, cytotoxicity assay, and counterimmunoelectrophoresis for the detection of Clostridium difficile and its toxin. Journal of Infectious Diseases, 147: 778.

Jewkes, J., Larson, H.E., Price, A.B., Sanderson, P.J. and Davies, H.A. (1981). The aetiology of acute diarrhoea in adults. Gut, 22: 388-392.

Johnson, T.A., Tabbut, B.R., and Page, C.O. (1981). Treatment of antibiotic-associated pseudomembranous colitis with metronidazole. American Journal of Hospital Pharmacy, 38: 1034-1035.

Justus, P.G., Martin, J.L., Goldberg, D.A., Taylor, N.S., Bartlett, J.G., Alexander, R.W. and Mathias, J.R. (1982). Myoelectric effects of Clostridium difficile: motility-altering factors distinct from its cytotoxin and enterotoxin in rabbits. Gastroenterology, 83: 836-843.

K

Kabins, S.A., and Spira, T.J. (1975). Outbreak of clindamycin-associated colitis. Annals of Internal Medicine, 83: 830-831.

Kappas, A., Shinagawa, N., Arabi, Y., Thompson, H., Burdon, D.W., Dimock, F., George, R.H., Alexander-Williams, J. and Keighley, M.R.B. (1978). Diagnosis of pseudomembranous colitis. British Medical Journal, 1: 675-678.

Katz, L., La Mont, J.T., Trier, J.S., Sonnenblick, E.B., Rothman, S.W., Broitman, S.A., and Rieth, S. (1978). Experimental clindamycin-association colitis in rabbits. Evidence for toxin-mediated mucosal damage. Gastroenterology, 74: 246-252.

Keighley, M.R.B., Burdon, D.W., Alexander-Williams, J., Shinagawa, N., Arabi, Y., Thompson, H., Youngs, D., Bentley, S. and George, R.H. (1978a). Diarrhoea and pseudomembranous colitis after gastrointestinal operations. A prospective study. The Lancet, ii: 1165-1167.

Keighley, M.R.B., Burdon, D.W., Arabi, Y., Alexander-Williams, J., Thompson, H., Youngs, D., Johnson, M., Bentley, S., George, R.H. and Mogg, G.A.G. (1978b). Randomised controlled trial of vancomycin for pseudomembranous colitis and postoperative diarrhoea. British Medical Journal, 2: 1667-1669.

Keighley, M.R.B., Arabi, Y., Alexander-Williams, J., Youngs, D., and Burdon, D.W. (1979a). Comparison between systemic and oral antimicrobial prophylaxis in colorectal surgery. The Lancet, i: 894-897.

Keighley, M.R.B., Burdon, D.W., Mogg, G.A.G., George, R.H., Alexander-Williams, J. and Thompson, H. (1979b). Pseudomembranous colitis. The Lancet, i: 559.

Keighley, M.R.B., Youngs, D., Johnson, M., Allan, R.N., and Burdon, D.W. (1982). Clostridium difficile toxin in acute diarrhoea complicating inflammatory bowel disease. Gut, 23: 410-414.

Kent, T.H. (1966). Staphylococcal enterotoxin gastroenteritis in Rhesus monkeys. American Journal of Pathology, 48: 387-407.

Kent, T.H., Formal, S.B., LaBree, E.H. and Takeuchi, A. (1966). Diffuse enteritis due to Salmonella typhimurium in opium-treated guinea pigs. Federation Proceedings, 25: 456.

Keusch, G.T., and Present, D.H. (1976). Summary of a workshop on clindamycin colitis. Journal of Infectious Diseases, 133: 578-587.

Keusch, G.T., and Donta, S.T. (1975). Classification of enterotoxins on the basis of activity in cell culture. The Journal of Infectious Diseases, 131: 58-63.

Kim, K-H., Fekety, R., Batts, D.H., Brown, D., Silva, J. Jr., and Waters, D. (1981). Isolation of Clostridium difficile from the environment and contacts of patients with antibiotic-associated colitis. Journal of Infectious Diseases, 143: 42-50.

King, C.Y., and Barriere, S.L. (1982). Analysis of the in vitro interaction between vancomycin and cholestyramine. Antimicrobial Agents and Chemotherapy, 19: 326-327.

King, G.S., and Murray, P.R. (1981). Ultrasctructural effects of Clostridium difficile cytotoxin on cultured cells. Abstracts of the Annual Meeting of the American Society for Microbiology, 1981: 22.

Kocandrle, V., Jouttuin, E., and Prohaska, J.V. (1966). Acute hemodynamic and gastrointestinal changes produced by staphylococcal exotoxin and enterotoxin in dogs. Journal of Surgical Research, 6: 50-57.

Koransky, J.R., Allen, S.D., and Dowell, V.R. (1978). Use of ethanol for selective isolation of spore forming microorganisms. Applied and Environmental Microbiology, 35: 762-765.

Kreutzer, E.W., and Milligan, F.D. (1978). Treatment of antibiotic-associated pseudomembranous colitis with cholestyramine resin. John Hopkins Medical Journal, 143: 67-72.

Kurkinen, M., Wartiovaara, J., and Vaheri, A. (1978). Cytochalasin B releases a major surface-associated glycoprotein, fibronectin, from cultured fibroblasts. Experimental Cell Research, 111: 127-137.

Kurzynski, T.A., Cembrowski, G.S., and Kimball, J.L. (1983). The use of CIE for the detection of Clostridium difficile toxin in stool filtrates: Laboratory and clinical correlation. American Journal of Clinical Pathology, 79: 370-374.

L

La Mont, J.T., Sonnenblick, E.B., Rothman, S. (1979). Role of clostridial toxin in the pathogenesis of clindamycin colitis in rabbits. Gastroenterology, 76: 356-361.

La Mont, J.T. and Trnka, Y.M. (1980). Therapeutic implications of Clostridium difficile toxin during relapse of chronic inflammatory bowel disease. The Lancet, i: 381-383.

Lory, S. and Collier, R.J. (1980). Diphtheria toxin: Nucleotide binding and toxin heterogeneity. Proceedings of the National Academy of Sciences, 77: 267-271.

Lowe, B.R., Onderdonk, A.B., and Bartlett, J.G. (1980). Abstracts of the American Society for Microbiology, C231, p.313.

Lowe, B.R., Fox, J.G., and Bartlett, J.G. (1980a). Clostridium difficile-associated cecitis in guinea pigs exposed to penicillin. American Journal of Veterinary Research, 41: 1277-1279.

Lusk, R.H., Fekety, F.R., Silva, J., Bodendorfer, T., Devine, B., Kawanishi, H., Korff, L., Nakauchi, D., Rogers, S., and Siskin, S.B. (1977). Gastrointestinal side effects of clindamycin and ampicillin therapy. Journal of Infectious Diseases, 135: (Suppl):S111-119.

Lusk, R.H., Fekety, R., Silva, J., Browne, R.A., Ringler, D.H., Abrams, G.D. (1978). Clindamycin-induced enterocolitis in hamsters. Journal of Infectious Diseases, 137: 464-475.

Lyerly, D.M., Lockwood, D.E., Richardson, S.H., and Wilkins, T.D. (1982). Biological activities of toxins A and B of Clostridium difficile. Infection and Immunity, 35: 1147-1150.

Lyerly, D.M., Sullivan, N.D.M., and Wilkins, T.D. (1983). Enzyme-linked immunosorbent assay for Clostridium difficile Toxin A. Journal of Clinical Microbiology, 17: 72-78.

M

McDonald, M., Ward, P., and Harvey, K. (1982). Antibiotic-associated diarrhoea and methicilllin-resistant Staphylococcus aureus. Medical Journal of Australia, 1: 462-464.

McKay, D.G., Hardaway, R.M., III, Wahle, G.H., Jr. and Hall, R.M. (1955). Experimental pseudomembranous enterocolitis: production by means of thrombosis of intestinal capillaries. Archives of Internal Medicine, 95: 779-787.

Madsen, G.L. and Knoop. F.C. (1981). Alteration of membrane permeability by Clostridium difficile toxin. Abstracts of the Annual Meeting of the American Society for Microbiology, 1981: 22.

Malamou-Ladas, H., and Tabaqchali, S. (1982). Inhibition by Clostridium difficile by faecal Streptococci. Journal of Medical Microbiology, 15: 569-574.

Marrie, T.J., Furlong, M., Faulkner, R.S., Sidorov, J., Haldane, E.V., and Kerr, E.A. (1982). Clostridium difficile: epidemiology and clinical features. Canadian Journal of Surgery, 25: 438-442.

Larson, H.E., Parry, J.V., Price, A.B., Davies, P.R., Dolby, J., and Tyrrell, D.A.J. (1977). Undescribed toxin in pseudomembranous colitis. British Medical Journal, 1: 1246-1248.

Larson, H.E., and Price, A.B. (1977). Pseudomembranous colitis: presence of clostridial toxin. The Lancet, 2: 1312-1314.

Larson, H.E., Price, A.B., Honour, P., and Borriello, S.P. (1978). Clostridium difficile and the aetiology of pseudomembranous colitis. The Lancet, 1: 1063-1066.

Larson, H.E. (1980). The experimental pathogenesis of antibiotic related colitis. Scandinavian Journal of Infectious Diseases, 22 (Supplement): 7-10.

Larson, H.E., Price, A.B., and Borriello, S.P. (1980). Epidemiology of experimental enterocecitis due to Clostridium difficile. Journal of Infectious Diseases, 142: 408-413.

Larson, H.E., Barclay, F.E., Honour, P., and Hill, I.D. (1982). Epidemiology of Clostridium difficile in infants. Journal of Infectious Diseases, 146: 727-733.

Lee, S.P., and Thomsen, L.L. (1982). Toxin-induced cell membrane injury in guinea pigs given lincomycin. Pathology, 14: 317-322.

Levine, H.G., Kennedy, M., and LaMont, J.T. (1982). Counterimmunoelectrophoresis vs. cytotoxicity assay for the detection of Clostridium difficile toxin. Journal of Infectious Diseases, 145: 398.

Levy, N.J., and Onderdonk, A.B. (1981). Lectin alterations of Clostridium difficile cytotoxin activity. Abstracts of the 21st ICAAC: 719.

Libby, J.M., Jortner, B.S., and Wilkins, T.D. (1982). Effect of the two toxins of C. difficile in the antibiotic-associated cecitis in hamsters. Infection and Immunity, 36: 822-829.

Libby, J.M., and Wilkins, T.D. (1982). Production of antitoxins to two toxins of Clostridium difficile and immunological comparison of the toxins by cross-neutralization studies. Infection and Immunity, 35: 374-376.

Libby, J., Donta, S., and Wilkins, T.D. (1983). Clostridium difficile toxin A in infants. Submitted for publication.

Lishman, A.H., Al-Jumaili, I.J., and Record, C.O. (1981a). Spectrum of antibiotic-associated diarrhea. Gut: 34-37.

Lishman, A., Al-Jumaili, I., and Record, C. (1981). Antitoxin production in antibiotic-associated colitis? Journal of Clinical Pathology, 34: 414-415.

Maxfield, F.R. (1982). Weak bases and ionophores rapidly and reversibly raise the pH of endocytic vesicles in cultured mouse fibroblasts. The Journal of Cell Biology, 95: 676-681.

Meyers, S., Mayer, L., Bottone, E., Desmond, E., and Janowitz, H.D. (1981). Occurrence of Clostridium difficile toxin during the course of inflammatory bowel disease. Gastroenterology, 80: 697-700.

Michelich, V.J., Nunez-Montiel, O., Schuster, G.S., Thompson, F., and Dowell, V.R. (1981). Diet as a coadjuvant for development of antibiotic-associated diarrhea in hamsters (Mesocricetus auratus). Laboratory Animal Science, 31: 259-262.

Middlebrook, J.L., and Dorland, R.B. (1979). Protection of mammalian cells from diphtheria toxin by exogenous nucleotides. Canadian Journal of Microbiology, 25: 285-290.

Middlebrook, J.L., Dorland, R.B. and Leppla, S.H. (1979). Effects of lectins on the interaction of diphtheria toxin with mammalian cells. Experimental Cell Research, 121: 95-101.

Middlebrook, J.L., and Kohn, L.D. eds. (1981). Receptor-mediated binding and internalization of toxins and hormones. Academic Press, New York.

Miranda, A.F., Godman, G.C. and Tanenbaum, S.W. (1974). Action of cytochalasin D on cells of established lines. The Journal of Cell Biology, 62: 406-423.

Mitchell, I.G., and Kenworthy, R. (1976). Investigations on a metabolite from Lactobacillus bulgaricus which neutralizes the effect of enterotoxin from Escherichia coli pathogenic for pigs. Journal of Applied Bacteriology, 41: 163-174.

Mogg, G.A.G., Keighley, M.R.B., Burdon, D.W., Alexander-Williams, J., Youngs, D., Johnson, M., Bentley, S., and George, R.H. (1979). Antibiotic-associated colitis - a review of 66 cases. British Journal of Surgery, 66: 738-742.

Mogg, G.A.G., Arabi, Y., Youngs, D., Johnson, M., Bentley, S., Burdon, D.W., and Keighley, M.R.B. (1980). Therapeutic trials of antibiotic-associated colitis. Scandinavian Journal of Infectious Diseases, 22: 41-45.

Mogg, G.A.G., George, R.H., Youngs, D., Johnson, M., Thompson, H., Burton, D.W., and Keighley, M.R.B. (1982). Randomized controlled trial of colestipol in antibiotic-associated colitis. British Medical Journal, 69: 137-139.

Moskovitz, M., and Bartlett, J.G. (1981). Recurrent pseudomembranous colitis unassociated with prior antibiotic therapy. Archives of Internal Medicine, 141: 663-664.

Mulligan, M.E., Rolfe, R.D., Finegold, S.M., George, W.L. (1979). Contamination of a hospital environment by Clostridium difficile. Current Microbiology, 3: 173-175.

Mulligan, M.E., Edelstein, M.A.C., and George, W.L. (1980a). Effect of cefoxitin therapy on fecal flora. In: Abstracts of the Annual Meeting of the American Society for Microbiology, 1980. American Society for Microbiology, Washington, D.C. Abstract A35, p.6.

Mulligan, M.E., George, W.L., Rolfe, R.D., and Finegold, S.M. (1980b). Epidemiological aspects of Clostridium difficile-induced diarrhea and colitis. American Journal of Clinical Nutrition, 33: 2533-2538.

Mulligan, M.E., Jeffes, L.E., Oishi, J.S., Blachman, U., Miranda, C. and Edelstein, M. (1982). Selective broth medium for Clostridium difficile. In: Abstracts of the Annual Meeting of the American Society for Microbiology, 1982, American Society for Microbiology, Washington, D.C., Abstract C301, p.321.

N

Nakamura, S., Mikawa, M., Nakshio, S., Takabatake, M., Okado, I., Yamakawa, K., Serikawa, T., Okumura, S., and Nishida, S. (1981a). Isolation of Clostridium difficile from the feces and the antibody in sera of young and elderly adults. Microbiology and Immunology, 25: 345-351.

Nakamura, S., Serikawa, T., Mikawa, M., Nakashio, S., Yamakawa, K., and Nishida, S. (1981b). Agglutination, toxigenicity and sorbitol fermentation of Clostridium difficile. Microbiology and Immunology, 25: 863-870.

Nash, J.Q., Chattopadhyay, B., Honeycombe, J. and Tabaqchali, S. (1982). Clostridium difficile and cytotoxin in routine faecal specimens. Journal of Clinical Pathology, 35: 561-565.

Nicolopoulos, N.G., Stathapoulos, E.N., Douzinas, E.E., and Vassilakis, J.S. (1981). Pseudomembranous colitis. Treatment by metronidazole. Hepato-Gastroenterology, 28: 120-122.

Nunez-Montiel, O.L., Thompson, F.S., and Dowell, V.R. (1983). Norleucine-tyrosine broth for rapid identification of Clostridium difficile by gas-liquid chromatography. Journal of Clinical Microbiology, 17: 382-385.

O

O'Connor, R.P., Silva, J., and Fekety, R. (1981). Rifampicin and antibiotic-associated colitis. Lancet, 1: 499.

Oishi, J.S., Mulligan, M.E., and Finegold, S.M. Failure to detect Clostridium difficile in foods. Journal of Infectious Diseases, (in press).

Onderdonk, A.B., Cisneros, R.L., and Bartlett, J.G. (1980). Clostridium difficile in gnotobiotic mice. Infection and Immunity, 28: 277-282.

Osborn, M., and Weber, K. (1977). The detergent-resistant cytoskeleton of tissue culture cells includes the nucleus and the mcirofilament bundles. Experimental Cell Research, 106: 339-349.

P

Pashby, N.L., Bolton, R.P. and Sherriff, R.J. (1979). Oral metronidazole in Clostridium difficile colitis. British Medical Journal, 1: 1605-1606.

Penner, A., Bernheim, A. (1939). Acute post-operative enterocolitis. Archives of Pathology, 27: 966-983.

Peikin, S.R., Galdibini, J., and Bartlett, J.G. (1980). Role of Clostridium difficile in a case of nonantibiotic-associated pseudomembranous colitis. Gastroenterology, 79: 948-951.

Pettet, J.D., Baggenstoss, A.H., Dearing, W.H., and Judd, E.S. (1954). Post-operative pseudomembranous enterocolitis. Surgery, Gynaecology and Obstetrics, 98: 546-552.

Phillips, K.D., and Rogers, P.A. (1981). Rapid detection and presumptive identification of Clostridium difficile by p-cresol production and selective medium. Journal of Clinical Pathology, 34: 642-644.

Piot, P., Stamm, W.E., Totten, P., and Holmes, K.K. (1980). Corynebacterium genitalium, Corynebacterium pseudogenitalium, Staphylococcus saprophyticus and Clostridium difficile in nongonococcal urethritis. In Third International Sexually Transmitted Diseases Meeting. International Society for Sexually Transmitted Diseases Research. Abstract 35.

Potuliege, C., Labbé, M. and Yourassowsky, E. (1981). Gas-liquid chromatography as screening test for Clostridium difficile. The Lancet, ii: 1105.

Poxton, I.R. (1982). Detection and isolation of Clostridium difficile. European Journal of Chemotherapy and Antibiotics, 2: 123-128.

Poxton, I.R. and Byrne, M.D. (1981a). Immunological analysis of the EDTA-soluble antigens of Clostridium difficile and related species. Journal of General Microbiology, 122: 41-46.

Poxton, I.R., and Byrne, M.D. (1981b). Detection of Clostridium difficile toxin by counterimmunoelectrophoresis: a note of caution. Journal of Clinical Microbiology, 14: 239.

Price, A.B., and Davies, D.R. (1977). Pseudomembranous colitis. Journal of Clinical Pathology, 30: 1-12.

Price, A.B., and Day, D.W. (1981). Pseudomembranous and infective colitis. In Recent Advances in Histopathology 11. ed. Anthony P.P., MacSween, R.N.M., Churchill Livingstone, Edinburgh, pp. 99-117.

Price, A.B., Jewkes, J., and Sanderson, P.J. (1979a). Acute diarrhoea: Campylobacter colitis and the role of rectal biopsy. Journal of Clinical Pathology, 32: 990-997.

Price, A.B., Larson, H.E., and Crow, J. (1979b). Morphology of experimental antibiotic-associated enterocolitis in the hamster: a model for human pseudomembranous colitis and antibiotic-associated diarrhoea. Gut, 20: 467-475.

R

Raibaud, P., Ducluzeau, R., Dubos, F., Hudault, S., Bewa, H. and Muller, M.C. (1980). Implantation of bacteria from the digestive tract of man and various animals into gnotobiotic mice. The American Journal of Clinical Nutrition, 33: 2440-2447.

Rampling, A., Warren, R.E., Berry, P.J., Swirsy, D., Hoggarth, C.E., and Bevan, P.C. (1982). Atypical *Clostridium difficile* colitis in neutropenic patients. The Lancet, ii: 162-163.

Rehg, J.E. (1980). Cecal toxin(s) from guinea pigs with clindamycin-associated colitis, neutralized by *Clostridium sordellii* antitoxin. Infection and Immunity, 27: 387-390.

Rehg, J.E., and Lu, Y-S. (1981). *Clostridium difficile* colitis in a rabbit following antibiotic therapy for Pasteurellosis. Journal of the American Veterinary Medical Association, 179: 1296-1297.

Rehg, J.E., and Lu, Y-S. (1982). *Clostridium difficile* typhlitis in hamsters not associated with antibiotic therapy. Journal of the American Veterinary Medical Association, 181: 1422-1423.

Rehg, J.E., and Pakes, S.P. (1982). Implication of *Clostridium difficile* and *Clostridium perfringens* iota toxins in experimental lincomycin-associated colitis in rabbits. Laboratory Animal Science, 32: 253-257.

Rehg, J.E., Yarbrough, B.A., and Pakes, S.P. (1980). Toxicity of cecal filtrates from guinea pigs with penicillin-associated colitis. Laboratory Animal Science, 30: 524-531.

Richardson, S.A., Brookfield, D.S.K., French, T.A. and Gray, J. (1981). Pseudomembranous colitis in a 5-week-old infant. British Medical Journal, 283: 1510.

Rietra, P.J.G.M., Slaterus, K.W., Zanen, H.C. and Meuwissen, S.G.M. (1978). Clostridial toxin in faeces of healthy infants. The Lancet, ii: 319.

Rifkin, G.D., Fekety, F.R., Silva, J., and Sack, R.B. (1977). Antibiotic-induced colitis. Implication of a toxin neutralised by Clostridium sordellii antitoxin. Lancet, ii: 1103-1106.

Rifkin, G.D., Fekety, R., and Silva, J. (1978a). Neutralization by Clostridium sordellii antitoxin of toxins implicated in clindamycin-induced cecitis in the hamster. Gastroenterology, 75: 422-424.

Rifkin, G.D., Silva, J., Jr., and Fekety, R. (1978b). Gastrointestinal and systemic toxicity of fecal extracts from hamsters with clindamycin-induced colitis. Gastroenterology, 74: 52-57.

Riley, T.U., and Karthigasu, K.T. (1982). Chronic osteomyelitis due to Clostridium difficile. British Medical Journal, 284: 1217-1218.

Rogers, T.R., Petrou, M., Lucas, C., Chung, J.T.N., Barrett, A.J., Borriello, S.P., and Honour, P. (1981). Spread of Clostridium difficile among patients receiving non-absorbable antibiotics for gut decontamination. British Medical Journal, 283: 408-409.

Rolfe, R.D., and Finegold, S.M. (1979). Purification and characterization of Clostridium difficile toxin. Infection and Immunity, 25: 191-201.

Rolfe, R.D., and Finegold, S.M. (1980). Inhibitory interactions between normal fecal flora and C. difficile. American Journal of Clinical Nutrition, 33: 2539.

Rolfe, R.D., and Finegold, S.M. (1983). Intestinal β-lactamase activity in ampicillin-induced, Clostridium difficile-associated ileocecitis. Journal of Infectious Diseases, 147: 227-235.

Rolfe, R.D., Halebian, S., and Finegold, S.M. (1981). Bacterial interference between Clostridium difficile and normal fecal flora. Journal of Infectious Diseases, 143: 470-475.

Rollins, D.E., and Moeller, D. (1976). Acute migratory polyarthritis associated with antibiotic-induced pseudomembranous colitis. American Journal of Gastroenterology, 65: 353-356.

Rossiter, K.A., Coulby, J., Wohlhieter, J.A., and Rothman, S.W. (1982). Isolation of plasmid DNA from toxigenic Clostridium difficile strains. Abstracts of the Annual Meeting of the American Society of Microbiology, Abst. 38.

Rothman, S.W. (1981). Presence of Clostridium difficile toxin in guinea pigs with penicillin-associated colitis. Medical Microbiology and Immunology, 169: 187-196.

Rothman, S.W., and Brown, J.E. (1981). Inhibition of membrane functions in intact HeLa cells by Clostridium difficile cytotoxic culture filtrates. Current Microbiology, 6: 221-224.

Rothman, S.W., Brown, J.E., Diecidue, A., and Foret, D. (1983). Differential cytotoxic effects of toxin A and toxin B isolated from Clostridium difficile. Federation Proceedings, 42: 1811 Abstract No. 317.

Ryan, R.W., Kwasnik, I., and Tilton, R.C. (1980). Rapid detection of Clostridium difficile toxin in human feces. Journal of Clinical Microbiology, 12: 776-779.

S

Sakurai, Y., Tsuchiya, H., Ikegami, F., Funatomi, T., Takasu, S., and Uchikoshi, T. (1979). Acute right-sided hemorrhagic colitis associated with oral administration of ampicillin. Digestive Diseases and Sciences, 24: 910-915.

Sanders, E. (1969). Bacterial interference I. Its occurrence among the respiratory tract flora and characterization of inhibition of Group A Streptococci by Viridan's Streptococci. Journal of Infectious Diseases, 120: 698-707.

Sanders, C.C., and Sanders, Jr., W.E. (1982). Enocin: an antibiotic produced by Streptococcus salivarius that may contribute to protection against infections due to group A Streptococci. Journal of Infectious Diseases, 146: 683-690.

Sands, M., Yungbluth, M., and Sommers, H.M. (1983). The non-value of counterimmunoelectrophoresis for the direct rapid detection of Clostridium difficile toxin in stool filtrates. American Journal of Clinical Pathology, 79: 375-377.

Schneider, D.L. (1981). ATP-dependent acidification of intact and disrupted lysosomes. Evidence for an ATP-driven proton pump. The Journal of Biological Chemistry, 256: 3858-3864.

Scopes, J.W., Smith, M.F., and Beach, R.C. (1980). Pseudomembranous colitis and sudden infant death. The Lancet, i: 1144.

Sell, T.L., Schaberg, D.R., and Fekety, R. (1982). Epidemiology of C. difficile infection: development of a bacteriophage and bacteriocin typing system. In: Abstracts of the Annual Meeting of the American Society for Microbiology, 1982. American Society for Microbiology, Washington, D.C., Abstract L26, p.86.

Sell, T.L., Schaberg, D.R., and Fekety, R. (1983). Bacteriophage and bacteriocin typing scheme for Clostridium difficile. Journal of Clinical Microbiology, 17: 1148-1152.

Seppala, K., Hjelt, L., and Sipponen, P. (1981). Colonoscopy in the diagnosis of antibiotic-associated colitis. A prospective study. Scandinavian Journal of Gastroenterology, 16: 465-468.

Shahani, K.M. and Ayebo, A.D. (1980). Role of dietary lactobacilli in gastrointestinal microecology. American Journal of Clinical Nutrition, 33: 2448-2457.

Sherertz, R.J., and Sarubbi, F.A. (1982). The prevalence of Clostridium difficile and toxin in a nursery population: a comparison between patients with necrotizing enterocolitis and an asymptomatic group. Journal of Pediatrics, 100: 435-439.

Silva, J. (1979). Animal models of antibiotic-induced colitis. In Schlessinger D. (ed.) Microbiology-1979. American Society for Microbiology, Washington, D.C., pp. 258-263.

Silva, J., Batts, D.H., Fekety, F.R., Plouffe, J., and Rifkin, G.D. (1980a). Successful treatment of clostridial colitis with oral vancomycin. In Current Chemotherapy and Infectious Diseases, American Society of Microbiology, pp. 957-958.

Silva, J., Lusk, R., Fekety, R., Wilson, K., Batts, D., Mason, D., and Spratt, D., (1980b). Immune responses of hamsters and humans with antibiotic-associated colitis. In Anaerobic Bacteria - Selected Topics. Lambe D.W., Genco, R.J., Mayberry-Carson, K.J. (eds), pp. 275-280.

Silva, J., Batts, D.H., Fekety, R., Plouffe, J.F., Rifkin, G.D., and Baird, I. (1981). Treatment of Clostridium difficile and diarrhea with vancomycin. American Journal of Medicine, 71: 815-822.

Small, J.D. (1968). Fatal enterocolitis in hamsters given lincomycin hydrochloride. Laboratory Animal Care, 18: 411-420.

Smith, C.J., Markowitz, S.M., and Macrina, F.L. (1981). Transferable tetracycline resistance in Clostridium difficile. Antimicrobial Agents and Chemotherapy, 19: 997-1003.

Smith, L.D.S., and King, E.O. (1962). Occurrence of Clostridium difficile in infections of man. Journal of Bacteriology, 84: 65-67.

Smith, M.F., Borriello, S.P., Claydon, G.S., and Casewell, M.W. (1980). Clinical and bacteriological findings in necrotising enterocolitis: a controlled study. Journal of Infection, 2: 23-31.

Snyder, M.L. (1937). Further studies of Bacillus difficilis (Hall and O'Toole). Journal of Infectious Diseases, 60: 223-231.

Stark, P.L., Lee, A., and Parsonage, B.D. (1982). Colonisation of the large bowel by Clostridium difficile in healthy infants : quantitative study. Infection and Immunity, 35: 895-899.

Stephen, J., and Pietrowski, R.A. (1981). Bacterial Toxins. Thomas Nelson and Sons Ltd., Surrey, pp. 26-33.

Sterne, M., and Wentzel, L.M. (1950). A new method for the large scale production of high-titre botulinum Formol-toxoid types C and D. Journal of Immunology, 65: 175-183.

Sullivan, N.M., Pellett, S., and Wilkins, T.D. (1982). Purification and characterization of toxins A and B of Clostridium difficile. Infection and Immunity, 35: 1032-1040.

Sullivan, N.M., and Wilkins, T.D. (1982). Production of Clostridium difficile-like toxins by Clostridium perfringens. Abstracts of the Annual meeting of the American Society for Microbiology. Abst. 37.

Sullivan, N.M., Lyerly, D.M., and Wilkins, T.D. (1983). Purification of Clostridium difficile toxin B and demonstration of multiple forms of the toxin. Submitted for publication.

Swartzberg, J.E., Maresca, R.M., and Remington, J.S. (1977). Clinical study of gastrointestinal complications associated with clindamycin therapy. Journal of Infectious Diseases, 135 (suppl):S99-103.

T

Takeda, Y., Takeda, T., Miwatani, T., and Ohtomo, N. (1978). Detection of cholera enterotoxin activity in suckling hamsters. Infection and Immunity, 19: 752-754.

Takeda, Y., Takeda, T., Yano, T., Yamamoto, K., and Miwatani, T. (1979). Purification and partial characterization of heat-stable enterotoxin of enterotoxigenic Escherichia coli. Infection and Immunity, 25: 978-985.

Taylor, N.S., and Bartlett, J.G. (1979). Partial purification and characterization of a cytotoxin from C. difficile. Reviews of Infectious Diseases, 1: 379-385.

Taylor, N.S., and Bartlett, J.G. (1980). Binding of Clostridium difficile cytotoxin and vancomycin by anion-exchange resins. Journal of Infectious Diseases, 141: 92-97.

Taylor, N.S., Onderdonk, A.B., and Bartlett, J.G. (1978). Partial purification and characterization of Clostridium difficile colitis toxin. 18th International Science Conference, Antimicrobial Agents and Chemotherapy, Abstract No. 127.

Taylor, N.S., Thorne, G.M., and Bartlett, J.G. (1980). Separation of an enterotoxin from the cytotoxin of Clostridium difficile. Clinical Research, 28: 285.

Taylor, N.S., Thorne, G.M., and Bartlett, J.G. (1981). Comparison of two toxins produced by Clostridium difficile. Infection and Immunity, 34: 1036-1043.

Tedesco, F.J. (1976). Clindamycin-associated colitis : review of the clinical spectrum of 47 cases. American Journal of Digestive Diseases, 21: 26-32.

Tedesco, F.J. (1979). Antibiotic-associated pseudomembranous colitis with negative proctosigmoidoscopy examination. Gastroenterology, 77: 295-297.

Tedesco, F.J. (1980). Bacitracin therapy in antibiotic-associated pseudomembranous colitis. Digestive Diseases and Sciences, 25: 783-784.

Tedesco, F.J. (1982a). Pseudomembranous colitis: pathogenesis and therapy. Medical Clinics of North America, 66: 655-664.

Tedesco, F.J. (1982b). Treatment of recurrent antibiotic-associated pseudomembranous colitis. American Journal of Gastroenterology, 77: 220-221.

Tedesco, F.J., Barton, R.W., and Alpers, D.H. (1974a). Clindamycin-associated colitis: a prospective study. Annals of Internal Medicine, 81: 429-433.

Tedesco, F.J., Stanley, R.J., and Alpers, D.H. (1974b). Diagnostic features of clindamycin associated pseudomembranous colitis. New England Journal of Medicine, 290: 841-843.

Tedesco, F., Gurwith, M., Markham, R., Christie, D., and Bartlett, J.G. (1978). Oral vanmycin for antibiotic-associated pseudomembranous colitis. The Lancet, II: 226-228.

Tedesco, F.J., Corless, J.K., and Brownstein, R.E. (1982). Rectal sparing in antibiotic-associated pseudomembranous colitis: a prospective study. Gastroenterology, 83: 1259-60.

Thelestam, M., and Bronnegard, M. (1979). Partial purification and cytotoxic effects of Clostridium difficile toxin. Toxicon, 17: 192.

Thelestam, M., Bronnegard, M. (1980). Interaction of cytopathogenic toxin from Clostridium difficile with cells in tissue culture. Scandinavian Journal of Infectious Diseases, Suppl. 22: 16-29.

Thelestam, M., and Möllby, R. (1975). Sensitive assay for detection of toxin-induced damage to the cytoplasmic membrane of human diploid fibroblasts. Infection and Immunity, 12: 225-232.

Thelestam, M., and Möllby, R. (1976). Cytotoxic effects on the plasma membrane of human diploid fibroblasts - a comparative study of leakage tests. Medical Biology, 54: 39-49.

Thelestam, M. and Möllby, R. (1983). Survival of cultured cells after functional and structural disorganization of plasma membrane by bacterial haemolysins and phospholipases. Toxicon, (in press).

Thomas, D.E.M., Fernie, D.S., Malone, M., Bayston, R., and Spitz, L. (1982). Association between Clostridium difficile and enterocolitis in Hirschsprung's disease. The Lancet, i: 78-79.

Toffler, R.B., Pingoud, E.G., and Burrell, M.I. (1978). Acute colitis related to penicillin and penicillin derivatives. The Lancet, ii: 707-709.

Toshniwal, R., Fekety, R., and Silva, J. (1979). Etiology of tetracycline-associated pseudomembranous colitis in hamsters. Antimicrobial Agents and Chemotherapy, 16: 167-170.

Toshniwal, R., Silva, J., Fekety, R., and Kim, K-H. (1981). Studies on the epidemiology of colitis due to Clostridium difficile in hamsters. Journal of Infectious Diseases, 143: 51-54.

Trnka, Y.M., and LaMont, J.T. (1981). Association of Clostridium difficile toxin with symptomatic relapse of chronic inflammatory bowel disease. Gastroenterology, 80: 693-696.

Tvede, M., and Willmsen, L. (1982). Clostridium difficile in patients with irritable bowel syndrome and ulcerative colitis. The Lancet, i: 1124.

V

Van Prohaska, J. (1959). Pseudomembranous enterocolitis. Archives of Surgery, 79: 197-206.

Van Prohaska, J., Jacobson, M.J., Drake, C.T., and Tan, T-L. (1959). Staphylococcus enterotoxin enteritis. Surgery, Gynecology and Obstetrics, 107: 73-77.

van der Waij, D., Berghuis, J.M., and Lekkerkerk, J.E.C. (1972). Colonization resistance of the digestive tract of mice during systemic antibiotic treatment. Journal of Hygiene, 70: 605-610.

Vesely, D.L., Straub, K.D., Nolan, C.M., Rolfe, R.D., Finegold, S.M., and Monson, T.P. (1981). Purified Clostridium difficile cytotoxin stimulates guanylate cyclase activity and inhibits adenylate cyclase activity. Infection and Immunity, 33: 285-291.

Vesely, D.L., Sullivan, N.M., Lyerly, D.M., Straub, D.D., Monson, T.P., and Wilkins, T.D. (1983). Clostridium difficile toxins A and B both enhance guanylate cyclase activity. Submitted for publication.

Viscidi, R.P., and Bartlett, J.G. (1981). Antibiotic-associated pseudomembranous colitis in children. Pediatrics, 67: 381-386.

Viscidi, R., Willey, S., and Bartlett, J.G. (1981). Isolation rates and toxigenic potential of Clostridium difficile isolates from various patient populations. Gastroenterology, 81: 5-9.

Viscidi, R., Yolken, R., Lauchon, B., Bo-Linn, P., Moench, T., and Bartlett, J.G. (1982). Serum antibody response to toxins A and B of Clostridium difficile. In: Program and Abstracts, 22nd Interscience Conference on Antimicrobial Agents and Chemotherapy, American Society for Microbiology, Washington, D.C. Abstract 595, p. 172.

W

Wada, N., Neshida, N., Iwaki, S., Ohi, H., Miyawaki, T., Taniguchi, N., and Migita, S. (1980). Neutralizing activity against Clostridium difficile toxin in the supernatants of cultured colostral cells. Infection and Immunity, 29: 545-550.

Wald, A., Mendelow, H., and Bartlett, J.G. (1980). Non-antibiotic associated pseudomembranous colitis due to toxin producing clostridia. Annals of Internal Medicine, 92: 798-799.

Walters, B.A.J., Stafford, R., Roberts, R.K., and Seneviraine, E. (1982). Contamination and cross-infection with Clostridium difficile in an intensive care unit. Australia and New Zealand and Journal of Medicine, 12: 255-258.

Wayne-Moss, C., and Nunez-Montiel, O.L. (1982). Analysis of short-chain acids from bacteria by gas-liquid chromatography with a fused-silica capillary column. Journal of Clinical Microbiology, 15: 308-311.

Weber, K., and Glenney, Jr., J.R. (1982). Calcium-modulated multifunctional proteins regulating F-actin organization. In Cold Spring Harbor Symposia on Quantitative Biology, volume XLV Cold Spring harbor Laboratory, pp. 541-552.

Wedel, N., Toselli, P., Pothoulakis, C., Faris, B., Oliver, P., Franzblau, C. and LaMont, T. (1983). Ultrastructural effects of Clostridium difficile toxin B on smooth muscle cells and fibroblasts. Experimental Cell Research, (in press).

Welch, D.F., Menge, S.K., and Matsen, J.M. (1980). Identification of toxigenic Clostridium difficile by counterimmunoelectrophoresis. Journal of Clinical Microbiology, 11: 470-473.

Welling, G.W., and Groen, G. (1978). β-Aspartylglycine, a substance unique to caecal contents of germfree and antibiotic-treated mice. Biochemical Journal, 175: 807-812.

Welling, G.W., Groen, G., Tuinte, J.H.M., Koopman, J.P. and Kennis, H.M. (1980). Biochemical effects on germ-free mice of association with several strains of anaerobic bacteria. Journal of General Microbiology, 117: 57-63.

Wells, C.L., Sugiyama, H. and Bland, S.E. (1982). Resistance of mice with limited intestinal flora to enteric colonization by Clostridium botulinum. Journal of Infectious Diseases, 146: 791-796.

Wessells, N.K., Spooner, B.S., Ash, J.F., Bradley, M.O., Luduena, M.A., Taylor, E.L. Wrenn, J.T., and Yamada, K.M. (1971). Microfilaments in cellular and developmental processes. Science, 171: 135-143.

West, S.E.H., and Wilkins, T.D. (1982). Problems associated with counter-immunoelectrophoresis assays for detecting Clostridium difficile toxin. Journal of Clinical Microbiology, 15: 347-349.

Wilkins, T.D. (1979). Discussion at symposium entitled "Virulence Factors of anaerobic bacteria", Boston, July 17-18, 1978. Reviews of Infectious Diseases, 1: 397.

Wilkins, T.D., Tsai, C.C., Aswell, J.E., Ehrich, M., Van Tassell, R.L., and Holdeman, L.V. (1978). Toxins of Clostridium difficile and C. sordellii. 18th International Science Conference, Antimicrobial Agents and Chemotherapy, Abstract, No. 437.

Wilkins, T., Ehrich, M., Van Tassell, R., and Balish, E. (1980). Studies on the clostridial toxin associated with antibiotic-associated pseudomembranous colitis. In Natural Toxins Eds. Eaker, D., and Wadstrom, T.), Pergamon Press, New York. pp. 411-417.

Willey, S., and Bartlett, J.G. (1979). Cultures for Clostridium difficile in stools containing a cytotoxin neutralized by Clostridium sordellii antitoxin. Journal of Clinical Microbiology, 10: 880-884.

Wilson, K.H., and Sheagren, J.N. (1983). Antagonism of toxigenic Clostridium difficile by nontoxigenic C. difficile. Journal of Infectious Diseases, 147: 733-736.

Wilson, K.H., Silva, J., and Fekety, R. (1980). Antagonism between the normal caecal flora of hamsters and C. difficile. Abstracts of the Interscience Conference on Antimicrobial Agents and Chemotherapy. Abstract 209.

Wilson, K.H., Silva, J., and Fekety, F.R. (1981). Suppression of Clostridium difficile by normal hamster cecal flora and prevention of antibiotic-associated cecitis. Infection and Immunity, 34: 626-628.

Wilson, K.H., Kennedy, M.J., Fekety, F.R. (1982a). Use of sodium taurocholate to enhance spore recovery on a medium selection for Clostridium difficile. Journal of Clinical Microbiology, 15: 443-446.

Wilson, K.H., Silva, J., and Fekety, F.R. (1982b). Fluorescent-antibody test for detection of Clostridium difficile in stool specimens. Journal of Clinical Microbiology, 16: 464-468.

Winans, L., Jr., Thornton, G.B., and Carski, T.R. (1980). The effect of Lactinex granules on Clostridium difficile induced pseudomembranous colitis. Abstracts of Annual Meeting American Society of Microbiology, Abstract A4

Wood, J.S., Bennett, I.L., and Yardley, J.H. (1956). Staphylococcal enterocolitis in chinchillas. Bulletin of the Johns Hopkins Hospital, 98: 454-463.

Wortmann, J., Prinz, R., Ullrich, K. and von Figura, K. (1979). Effect of lectins on the metabolism of sulfated glycosaminoglycans in cultured fibroblasts. Biochimica et Biophysica Acta, 588: 26-34.

Wu, A. (1982). Spontaneous persistent pseudomembranous colitis related to Clostridium difficile in ischaemic bowel disease. British Medical Journal, i: 1606-1607.

Wu, T.C., and Fung, J.C. (1983). Evaluation of the usefulness of counterimmunoelectrophoresis for diagnosis of Clostridium difficile - associated colitis in clinical specimens. Journal of Clinical Microbiology, 17: 610-613.

Wüst, J., Sullivan, N.M., Hardegger, U., and Wilkins, T.D. (1982). Investigation of an outbreak of antibiotic-associated colitis by various typing methods. Journal of Clinical Microbiology, 16: 1096-1101.

Y

Yolken, R.H., Whitcomb, L.S., Marien, G., Bartlett, J.G., Libby, J., Ehrich, M., and Wilkins, T. (1981). Enzyme Immunoassay for the detection of Clostridium difficile antigen. Journal of Infectious Diseases, 144: 378.

www.ingramcontent.com/pod-product-compliance
Ingram Content Group UK Ltd.
Pitfield, Milton Keynes, MK11 3LW, UK
UKHW020819290926
15470UKWH00003B/1261
9780898386233